She is not your rehab

One man's journey to healing and the global anti-violence movement he inspired.

MATT BROWN
with SARAH BROWN

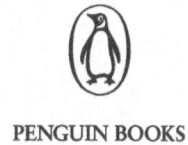

PENGUIN BOOKS

PENGUIN

UK | USA | Canada | Ireland | Australia
India | New Zealand | South Africa | China

Penguin is an imprint of the Penguin Random House group of companies,
whose addresses can be found at global.penguinrandomhouse.com.

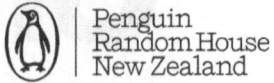

First published by Penguin Random House New Zealand, 2021

1 3 5 7 9 10 8 6 4 2

Text © Matt Brown and Sarah Brown, 2021

The moral right of the authors has been asserted.

All rights reserved. Without limiting the rights under copyright
reserved above, no part of this publication may be reproduced,
stored in or introduced into a retrieval system, or transmitted,
in any form or by any means (electronic, mechanical, photocopying,
recording or otherwise), without the prior written permission of both
the copyright owner and the above publisher of this book.

Cover design by Katrina Duncan © Penguin Random House New Zealand
Text design by Carla Sy © Penguin Random House New Zealand
Cover and internal photographs by Jared Yeoward
Prepress by Image Centre Group
Printed and bound in Australia by Griffin Press, an Accredited
ISO AS/NZS 14001 Environmental Management Systems Printer

A catalogue record for this book is available from
the National Library of New Zealand.

ISBN 978-0-14-377598-0
ISBN (audio) 978-0-14-377655-0
eISBN 978-0-14-377599-7

penguin.co.nz

The assistance of Ministry of Social Development Te Manatū Whakahiato Ora
towards the production of this book is gratefully acknowledged by the publisher.

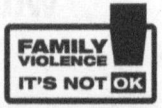

Except for historical figures, and my and my wife's names,
the names of people who feature in this book and the case
studies have been altered to protect their privacy.

The information contained in this book is of a general nature only and not a substitute for professional medical advice. If you wish to make any use of information in this book relating to your health, you should first consider its appropriateness to your situation and obtain advice from a medical professional.

I WROTE THIS BOOK on behalf of every kid who ever lived in a home of violence and abuse. The ones who had all their dreams kicked out of them. I wrote this for you. Because I am you.

And I'm here to say that it's possible to change the narrative. It's possible to eventually be everything we never got.

I'm living proof that a kid raised in violence and abuse for the first 15 years of his life can dream of being something else.

And then *be* something else.

And I wrote this book in honour of my Mum.

But more than dedicating all the words on these pages to you, I dedicate my life, in honour of you, Mum, to healing. In the hope that anyone who reads this book may find some insight into the prevention of the sad eyes you carried every day of the life that we shared. Those eyes - your eyes - were imprinted onto my spirit.

I love you and I look forward to the day you embrace and lecture me again.

May your memory be a revolution.

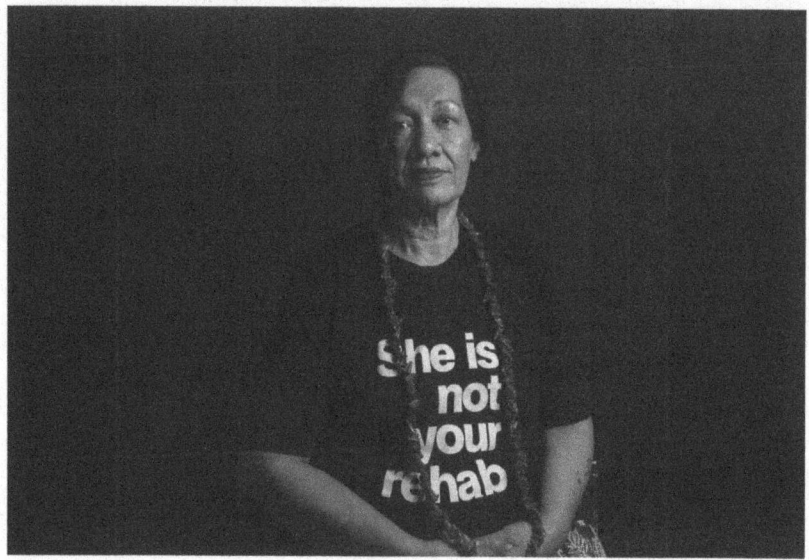

Contents

Before we begin 9

A note on self-care 13

In a little tin-shed barbershop in the hood ... 15

Chapter one: She is not your rehab 25

Chapter two: She is not your mother 45

Chapter three: She is not your absent father 61

Chapter four: She is not your shame 79

Chapter five: She is not your trauma 93

Chapter six: She is not your saviour 107

Chapter seven: She is not your ex 121

Chapter eight: She is not auditioning for you 133

Chapter nine: She is not your porn star 145

Chapter ten: She is not your prison 159

Chapter eleven: She is not your lifeline 175

Chapter twelve: She is not your hired help 189

Chapter thirteen: She is not your punching bag 203

Chapter fourteen: She is not yours to control 219

Chapter fifteen: She is not your doormat 233

Chapter sixteen: She is not your competition 245

Chapter seventeen: She is not your bank account 257

Chapter eighteen: She is not your quick fix 269

Chapter nineteen: She is not your trophy 283

Chapter twenty: She is not your grief 293

Chapter twenty-one: She is not your excuse 303

An invitation to heal 313

Acknowledgements 316

Quotations and Resources 319

About the author 320

Before we begin

I WRITE IN DEDICATION and gratitude for every single man who has ever sat in my barbershop. This book is in honour of you. This book is in gratitude for our conversations, our laughs and our tears. I count those as the trophies of my barbering career I am most proud of.

Many of you were born to Mothers who survived more than thrived, and Fathers who, sadly, never showed up for you in quite the way you needed; because they truly didn't know how to even show up for themselves. Because of this, so many of us weren't adequately loved or nurtured in the ways we so desperately desired and needed. Some of you could easily be dead after all you have endured.

My heart is with you, Brothers. I see you and acknowledge your pain. There are generations of abuse and trauma that have moulded and conditioned you into the men you are today. If only we could have a greater understanding of generational trauma: that you can take the child out of the trauma, but it can take years to take the trauma out of the child.

So I take this moment to be with each of you, my beloved Brothers. For just existing, when many times you may not have wanted to do even that. The journey has been long and arduous, and I thank you for choosing to still be with us.

Please understand that this book takes you how you are, where you are, but my desire is, ultimately, that it moves you further on your journey.

Changing you is not my goal and not my job; change is the inevitable outcome of real growth, so I hope this book *grows* you and your capacity to make lasting change for yourself, and for your future generations. I have found that there really are no successful quick fixes.

'There is no judgement here because, after years of talking with men of all ages and nationalities, I have been privileged to see underneath the hardest of exteriors, behind masks of all shapes and sizes, to see a side of men that is so raw and beautiful. We were each born to love and be loved. I haven't met a man yet who doesn't, at the deepest level, desire this for his life.'

I believe that the nature of life is that we are either growing or dead, and I have personally encountered many men who are like the walking dead, merely just existing.

This book, I hope, brings life into the places inside you that have been dead for longer than you care to admit. I pray that the insights found here are helpful in your journey to healing and wholeness.

I will keep it real, black and white, straight to the point, as I know us men prefer.

This is a book for you.

But this book is also for me. It's the book I wish I'd had when I started my path of healing. So I write all this to me, too, as a reminder.

There is no judgement here because, after years of talking with men of all ages and nationalities, I have been privileged to see underneath the hardest of exteriors, behind masks of all shapes and sizes, to see a side of men that is so raw and beautiful. We were each born to love and be loved. I haven't met a man yet who doesn't, at the deepest level, desire this for his life.

She Is Not Your Rehab is written simply because no other living person can be - or do - that for us. The price is much too high and comes at too great a cost. Our healing cannot come at the expense of our life partner's, and all too often I have seen that approach - where men dump their problems on their women - and it fails. It fails because it's too big a burden to pass on to someone else. Her wellbeing, and her own journey into healing, can't take that extra load. And it's not hers to take.

In my years of barbering I have listened intently to the men in my chair, and I have truly heard the pain of a collective broken heart.

This book is my response.

A note on self-care

BEFORE WE GO ANY FURTHER, let's take a moment to pause and reflect on what we are about to do, and how best to do it lovingly and safely. For, my Brothers (and Sisters, if you're reading this), as we go on this journey together - sharing my story and searching for your own best new path - we will be encountering experiences and subjects that might trigger strong emotions and feelings and memories. And just as much as this book is about us taking personal responsibility for our lives and actions, it is also about us finding support and community. So while only you can do the learning and growing, those who love you can support you and walk by your side. And, as the book will also show you, sometimes that support is best provided by a professional or someone with experience of how these personal journeys are made.

So if some of the things we talk about are triggering for you and you need to talk, please reach out. Part of our journey, after all, is about learning how to talk about the painful things inside us.

I have included the contact information for some places in New Zealand that can provide support on page 319 of this book.

In a little tin-shed barbershop in the hood...

GROWING UP IN CHRISTCHURCH, New Zealand, I witnessed many things a child should never have to experience. I saw constant hurt, pain and ongoing abuse being inflicted on everyone I loved. I, too, was a recipient of this violence. I didn't have the words then to explain what I saw happening, and I didn't even really realise this life wasn't normal – that other people didn't experience or endure what we had to live with.

To me, it was all I knew.

I grew up in a three-bedroom state house, with my four New Zealand-born brothers (I am the middle of five boys) and three older half-sisters who came over from Sāmoa to live with us at different points later in life. Our baby sister Katherine died at birth, and while our parents came to New Zealand from Sāmoa for a better life, to say they struggled to get that 'better life' is an understatement. Our parents spent their entire lives working in factories for very low wages, and we lived as poor as you could in a modern New Zealand context.

Dad was an alcoholic and would beat my Mother regularly

– at least weekly – but often the cycle of physical violence and emotional abuse was a daily occurrence, so that it seemed like an endless experience for us all.

We had an 'open home', which meant all kinds of people would come in and out of our house constantly, and that resulted in multiple incidents of sexual abuse by relatives and associates.

My love of art and music was my refuge. The nineties hip-hop scene, and Tupac Shakur in particular, gave me an outlet that I connected deeply with. The music room at my high school became my safe space, and my music teacher let me hide out there after school, so I could temporarily delay going home and having to face what was happening there.

Home for me never ever felt safe.

'Being a barber, I have come to understand the extraordinary gift my job is, and the power I have to challenge an often-negative narrative that society has about men.'

It was also music that brought my wife Sarah into my life, but you'll find out more about our journey of awakening to love together throughout this book, because our story has made me understand how relationships can either help or hinder your healing. How, at the end of the day, each one of us needs to sort our own shit out!

I've been a barber now for over a decade. Because of my history, when I first started my barbershop I wanted it to be more than just a barbershop. Prior to being a barber, I was a joiner by trade. Then one day I woke up and decided that a hobby I'd had since high school – barbering – could actually be a job, *and* a way I could connect with the men in my neighbourhood. The reality was no one was coming for us. So yes, I wanted to give dope fades, like those of the hip-hop stars I so admired, but I also wanted my barbershop to be more of a place where men could be seen.

I wanted to connect on a deeper level with guys I knew from the hood, guys I had grown up with. I knew first-hand the power of a haircut - and how it could change the way we feel about ourselves inside. I thought if I could combine a great haircut with a listening ear, then maybe something special could happen.

So many of the guys in my neighbourhood had gone down paths of joining gangs, becoming incarcerated or addicted, with some even tragically ending their lives. I saw pain all across my community.

And I knew why. The sad truth is that while many of us were now out in the real world, we were still traumatised from the childhoods we had barely survived, and were coping however we could. Their stories were my stories, and my stories were theirs.

It was our pain that made us a family. Inside my very first tin-shed barbershop, which I started in my backyard, we'd laugh together about the hidings we got as kids, or how our Mothers would gamble away the food money on Thursdays, or how many times our Fathers had been inside prison. It wasn't funny at all, but somehow these conversations kept us all from not feeling alone in our pain.

Shared pain somehow feels less traumatic.

I could call these men my first clients, but, really, they became so much more. They were my friends, my Brothers, my teachers - more than that, they were my insight into humanity.

I started to spend my days, and many nights, talking to the men in my city. They were all ages, and from all walks of life. We talked about their deeper pain, their untold stories, and the things they regretted or wanted to change. So funnily enough it was in that barbershop - with me mostly looking at the back of their heads - where they felt the most seen, they told me.

Those early conversations were special, and I'll never forget the very first time, after deeply connecting with a client who was experiencing suicidal thoughts, when I thought: 'This is it! My job here, in my garden-shed barbershop in the hood, could make an actual difference in people's lives!' This moment forever changed my barbering career, because every day, as I'm cleaning my tools and getting ready for my day, I know, without doubt, that I can make a difference by genuinely seeing and hearing the men who sit in my chair.

The truth is there are ways we can all impact our communities, and become part of changing a culture in positive ways to universally raise consciousness. We can each redefine what 'traditional masculinity' looks like in whatever job we do. Being a barber, I have come to understand the extraordinary gift my job comes with, and the power I have to challenge an often-negative narrative that society has about men.

Not many people are allowed into another man's personal space quite like a barber is, and for that reason I consider the work I do as sacred. Barbering, to me, is an authentic journey of men. It's learning to accept a man exactly as he comes to me in my chair, and serving him without judgement. Only then can I see the beauty in the men hiding behind the masks that, often, they have nowhere else to remove.

In this book, I will introduce you to the people and the concepts that have helped me on my own journey of healing. These ideas may work for you, or they may not, but I invite you to begin your journey of healing now. There is never a better time than now, and if you ever needed one, this is your invitation.

What you read here may spark ideas that take you on a completely different path to mine, and that's okay, as long as you're willing to take responsibility for your own feelings and actions. I don't believe in a 'one size fits all' approach to healing, because we are each so unique in our experiences and personalities that the path for each of us will inevitably be as varied as we are.

I wouldn't call myself a scholar by any stretch, but I'm an avid learner, and a student of life, and when I genuinely seek wisdom and understanding, I find my teachers in the most unexpected forms. When I first discovered Dr Brené Brown (who I jokingly call my 'white Mama', and who has no idea she has a Sāmoan son), she taught me so much about vulnerability and shame, courage and empathy, that it was like a lightbulb inside of me immediately switched on and stayed on. My eyes and my heart were suddenly aware of all the things I didn't know I had experienced in my life – what a gift to my awareness and life her teaching was.

Simply, I had learnt a whole new language for my experiences, which profoundly affected my own healing journey and consciousness in my work with men, who often wouldn't think they could learn anything from a white lady from Texas. I'd attempt to take her insight and ideas, and translate them into language that resonates with us; the Brothers in my neighbourhood. This is what I aspire to do in this book, too. I have learnt so many things from all kinds of sources along my path, and have found that there is simplicity in those teachings. Because the truth is, my Brothers, that there is a profound yet simple truth and frequency that we all understand, and relate to on a deep level. We can learn anywhere and from anyone; our humanity connects us all, and what comes from the heart always reaches the heart.

I've learnt about 'love languages', which taught me clearly how we each give and want to receive love from others. Dr Gary Chapman has identified five different 'love languages': acts of service; words of affirmation; gifts; quality time; and physical touch. Knowing about the different love languages has helped me (and many men I have shared it with in my barber's chair) be aware of how I prefer someone to show me love. I've even received bottles of wine from grateful wives because their husbands finally spoke their language! My wife Sarah's love language is 'words of affirmation' – hearing them makes her know she is loved; while mine is 'acts of service' – all the little things done for me show me I am loved. Once we had identified what these were, we were able to connect with each other deeply in ways that are meaningful to us.

Across cultures, ages and genders we can teach and learn from each other if we are prepared to seek to understand, rather than merely be understood.

Another thing Queen Brené and I have in common is being

invited to speak at a TEDx talk in our region. I was invited to speak at TEDxChristchurch in 2019 by my friend Kaila, and it gave me an opportunity to talk about the work we have done over the past 10 years in my barbershop with a completely different audience. It wasn't comfortable getting up in front of more than 2000 people and being open and vulnerable with my story. Prior to giving the talk, I asked my wife if an audience like that would even be interested in a story about a boy from the hood. She assured me that not only was my story worth sharing, but that it would resonate with people from all walks of life.

As I walked on stage I remembered thinking that all I actually had to do was be myself and own my story. There were tears along with laughs as the longest 18 minutes of my life sped by. We ended with a haka that myself, my wife and a client named Komene, who has become a Brother, wrote together. The words of our haka reflect the purpose of all of our work in the fight against violence. The feeling absolutely resounded around the building that night, and the energy or the wairua in that room was incredible.

DISCOVERING FORGIVENESS WAS HUGE for me, and is something I choose to do every single day. But forgiveness for me couldn't be that tokenistic ritual often preached at church in my early days, where it was taught as a way to essentially cover up abuse and condone bad behaviour. Rather, it had to be something that actually *worked*. It had to bring me *real* freedom.

For me, forgiveness became not a one-time event, but a whole practice of being forgiving and subsequently living with forgiveness. Throughout this book, I offer some of the strategies that I have learnt in my own journey – and sometimes it's as simple as speaking kindly with understanding to the little boy inside me who still longs to be heard, because nobody else knew how to do that when Little Matt was growing up.

I write about things like intergenerational trauma, and how hurt people in turn inevitably hurt other people. Pain demands to be felt, and it either manifests itself in things like self-hatred, self-harm, addictions or suicidal ideation, or in the ways we interact with those around us – in ways like family violence, bullying, and controlling and manipulative behaviour. These are all symptoms of pain within that must be healed.

If you were anything like me, and grew up with hurt parents who then manifested their hurt onto you, there will be a pain and a sadness that has existed in you for a long, long time. So long that you probably don't know how to feel any other way.

I'm here to tell you that now is the time to address that pain and sadness.

'If you were anything like me, and grew up with hurt parents who then manifested their hurt onto you, there will be a pain and a sadness that has existed in you for a long, long time. So long that you probably don't know how to feel any other way.'

Now is the time to learn a new way of thinking, and of being. Now is the time to heal.

It is totally possible to be something else, and by doing something new you're bravely breaking the cycle and changing the way your brain operates, and you're healing your family line for future generations to come. **Cycles repeat until one person has the courage to say: 'This shit stops with me.'**

This takes time, and dedication, but it is so worth persevering with and investing this time into your healing. No one else can do that for you.

So, maybe for the first time ever, you've decided that it is time for you.

I want you to know that you can do this, because I know that, without doubt, we each have the power to change abusive and traumatic family narratives, and be something different; we can be *more* than we ever received.

Since I started in my tin-shed barbershop, my life has changed in so many ways. It changed firstly because I have relentlessly been committed to my own healing, and actively sought insights that could lead to awareness and changed behaviour. No one else could do that for me.

I have surrounded myself with so many good men in my work, and have learnt so much about what healthy reciprocal relationships can actually be like. Just because I never saw that growing up, it in no way means I can't learn how to have one now in my own marriage. I changed the minute I realised I could change if I chose to. I realised I had to put the work into healing myself, and, while it took time and considerable effort, it is so

'I want you to know that you can do this, because I know that, without doubt, we each have the power to change abusive and traumatic family narratives, and be something different; we can be *more* than we ever received.'

worth it when I tuck my children in at night, and marvel that they lead a childhood nothing like mine. My children are safe with me, and I am proud that I broke the cycle of abuse for them.

The safe space we created in my barbershop has now been introduced into other barbershops and salons around Australasia, in prisons and indigenous communities, where talking about your feelings has not always been encouraged. I offer my teaching often in the form of wānanga and gatherings, collaborating alongside a number of other organisations in the social services sector, bringing this vital work into new places with men who have desperately needed the support and empathy that only a compassionate community can offer. I believe deeply that there is great power in collective healing when we do this work together.

This book can be a safe companion to help you examine your life without judgement, so you, too, can make the changes you need.

Show up for yourself today, Brother.

The journey of healing starts here.

Chapter one

She is not your rehab

MEN HAVE COME TO HER for many generations now, in a mixture of great desperation and relief. We've been unloading our baggage, like we're at the airport terminal and she's the carousel on which we can dump our stuff, so that we can then attempt to jet off in our life, hands-free.

When we expect her to be our rehab, all we have really done is transfer to her a burden that is not hers to bear, meaning she's struggling alone to carry not only her own burden but ours as well.

I see her so clearly; a woman walking through life literally weighed down, clinging onto other people's baggage, unable to move much at all. Then, by some miracle, she manages to somehow take a few steps forward, only to find more bags are being dumped on her by whoever she is with, causing her to eventually physically collapse. And all the while she has been denied the time and the energy to focus on her own growth and journey, to be the best she can be. The very experiences and traumas she carries with her, which may have convinced her that she needs to take on your burden, will not be healed. She is trapped. And so are you. There are no winners.

I know this woman well and picture her easily, because she is the Mother from my childhood.

But she is also any woman who has taken on too much in order to ease the load of others. And sadly, there are so many women who have done just that - perhaps most often for their intimate partners.

REHAB – THE SHORT WORD for rehabilitation - is the action of restoring something that has been damaged back to its former condition. The former condition is who any of us *really* are.

The boy inside you - the boy prior to any abuse, abandonment, humiliation, shame, betrayal or loss that you've experienced, and before all the suffering that this has brought you - he's still in there. We've each had our individual hurts that too often we have buried deep inside us, hoping that if we ignore them for long enough they will somehow disappear.

Throughout this book I want to speak to 'him' and call him forward.

Because he is who you really are, Brother. He is me. He is us.

We're in this together, and if you have ever felt alone in your pain, then this is where I'm here to gently remind you of the truth - that you are far from alone. Men all over the world struggle with not knowing where to start in their healing journey; I know this because over the past decade I have listened to all kinds of men sitting in my barber's chair, and so many feel alone about the things every other man feels!

But that boy, currently sitting at the age he was at the time of the trauma, still wants answers. He still longs to feel. He still needs someone to show up for him.

But what does 'showing up' even look like? For me, after a lifetime of disappointment, I didn't believe anyone would actually show up for me because, quite honestly, I was always being let down and disappointed. To avoid this, I expected nothing, and refused to ask anyone to do anything for me. That saved me so much heartache, I thought. But then I learnt how to

actually show up for myself in brand-new ways. I started small. I kept promises to myself – small things, like telling myself I would drink 3 litres of water a day, and then actually drinking the 3 litres. Then I'd move on to harder things like enforcing a boundary, and telling someone 'No' without justifying it or explaining my decision. These little things were instrumental in helping me to believe that I could show up for myself – that I had my own back like no one had before.

'This cemented hurt sits like a heavy weight in our hearts. And when someone gets close enough to this hardened, yet tender, heart of ours, it's in such a damaged state that it's easy to react rather than to respond when our old feelings are triggered. We want love and acceptance; we respond with hurt and rejection.'

Think about when something goes wrong – like you get a flat tyre, or you need help moving something big. Who do you call? Who shows up to help you? Wouldn't it be someone you know who would not only take your call, but would be in a position to help you – or at minimum suggest someone who can do what you ask? It may sound different, but **you can learn to be trustworthy and show up for yourself.**

If you are anything like me, and lived a childhood where people didn't show up for you, you now have to accept that, as painful as it is, they just didn't know how. They didn't know how to do it for themselves, so they couldn't show you or teach you how to show up for yourself.

And it's all these hurts – a lifetime of pain – that ultimately often bring us, without our even knowing, to seek rehabilitation in *her*, the woman in our life who we suddenly want to fix everything in us that hurts.

I say 'without our even knowing', because we don't realise that, deep down, we are reaching out for the love and acceptance we never felt. In fact, we act just the opposite – we push her away. Because those hidden hurts have not magically disappeared at all. In fact, the years of hiding have only cemented the bitterness and the agony that come from carrying a heavy burden around for way too long. This cemented hurt sits like a heavy weight in our hearts. And when someone gets close enough to this hardened, yet tender, heart of ours, it's in such a damaged state that it's easy to react rather than to respond when our old feelings are triggered. We want love and acceptance; we respond with hurt and rejection.

This is illustrated in a letter I received from a Brother who was struggling in the Covid-19 lockdown:

Dear Matt,

This lockdown is doing my head in.

I feel like a caged animal and things aren't going too well with the Mrs either. I read something you said about sitting with your anger so I did that last night.

I sat there while she was nagging on at me and wanted to throw something at her to shut her the fuck up, but instead went outside for a smoke, still fucked off. Tried to calm down and actually thought about why I hate being stuck here at home so much.

I thought about when I was younger my Mum's asshole boyfriend at the time would lock me in the laundry cupboard when he thought I was being a little shit. He hated me being around. I'd be in there for hours, even falling asleep or pissing myself sometimes. It was hot and cramped and I hated it. He didn't give a fuck, and if I cried or made any noise he'd make me stay there longer.

I never understood why Mum wouldn't come and get me out. I was only about 6 or 7 years old at the time, just a small kid!

Years later she told me she thought it was the safest place for me, away from him. I thought a lot about that last night, and I guess I'm writing to ask you what I should do in these times of frustration. I don't want to be an asshole to her, but honestly I see red when I feel cornered or nagged at.

Help, Bro. I just want to be free.

IN NEW ZEALAND, we had to go into Level 4 lockdown at the end of March 2020 for four weeks to battle the Covid-19 pandemic. This meant many people had to stay home, and only essential workers were allowed to go to work. It was a time of huge stress and uncertainty for all sorts of people – both men and women, young and old. I tried my best to respond to the many letters I received in my inbox from men who were struggling to live with themselves in this new reality. Here's what I wrote to the Brother whose letter is included above:

Dear Brother,

First of all thank you so much for your message.

Thank you for sharing a bit of your childhood with me. I'm so proud of you, for having the strength to sit there in your anger and allow the child within you who was once locked up to begin to have a voice.

I have experienced that very feeling of being dismissed/shut out/shut down and locked up. I've learnt the caged life has a look, a feel and a sound.

If you take a wild animal, throw it into the zoo/lock it up/put it behind bars, that animal will stalk in frustration with an instinct of survival/attack and escape. But over time, the animal becomes resigned, moves toward the back of the cage, angry and frustrated. The animal looks out into the world and resigns itself to a life of anger and frustration.

You can tell when a person is there because they have a recurring pattern of resignation and constant frustration. When they look at the world, they often point in anger and say: 'No one understands me at all!' And often, when the closest person to them offers help with the best intention for their wellbeing, they quickly roll their eyes with the thought: 'Stop nagging me, for fuck's sake.'

I was Mr 'Roll My Eyes' all the time in the beginning of my relationship, Brother. Whenever my wife would offer help or advice, or remind me to do something I said I was going to do but had procrastinated on, my eyes would go rolling, as would my thoughts. 'Who is she to tell me?' I'd think.

The ones we allow to love us the most will always trigger our most painful childhood memories, because there aren't many we allow close enough in to affect us in this way. While most of our hurts do come from relationships, so does our healing.

To apply that love and healing does take some work. Sitting in your anger and recognising your childhood pain, why you get frustrated easily when you feel trapped, is a beautiful first step, Brother.

I have this question for you: Do you believe your partner loves you?

If you do, then applying love and choosing the path of healing in this area of your life looks like telling yourself and your inner little boy this new truth.

Coach yourself and tell yourself this daily:

1. Life is better when you work from the belief that everyone is doing the best they can (including your Mother and your partner).

2. She (your partner) is not your Mother. As children we have a very minimal descriptive language for our feelings. We remember things but don't interpret them well. Society has taught us that mothers should be nurturing and protective of their babies. You didn't feel this locked in the cupboard, but Mum has now told you she thought she was trying to protect you. Believe that she did the best she could with what she knew at the time. Forgive her for not showing up for you how you needed then, and stop taking out the frustration you had with Mum then on the woman in your life now.

3. You are no longer that little boy stuck in the cupboard, but now a Man/Father/Partner who is responsible for your own healing and future. Do you want to stay a moment longer than you need to in the cupboard of fear/anger/frustration/rage? You can let yourself out of this cupboard now, Brother, by showing up for yourself in a new way. The lock is on the inside now, and you, Brother, are the one with the key.

4. If you believe your partner has the best intentions for you, then allowing her input/say/authority in your life will only add to your wellbeing, not take away from it.

5. There's a way for you to communicate your frustration effectively without resorting to physical or verbal violence. This looks like learning to enter into negotiation with her by expressing how you feel and learning to also keep your word with things you've said you'll do.

> Today, Brother, I want to whakamana you and tell you that I see you. I see the six-year-old boy sitting alone in that hot cupboard. I want him to know that someone is coming for him.
>
> That someone is you, Brother.
>
> You are learning to show up for yourself.
>
> It's new, but if you can free your mind and heart of this burden, I promise you it won't matter how long you'll be physically confined anywhere ... because you'll be free.
>
> Matt

I BELIEVE THE BOY inside you desires for you to be the man he once needed so badly to show up for him. That boy still needs you – in fact, he needs you to show up now like never before. We can all begin to do that for ourselves by learning to **be present with the pain inside ourselves** that often has never even been acknowledged, let alone felt enough to be helpful to us on our journey.

Through my own journey I've learnt that my pain has actually been the biggest invitation to heal. My pain is actually a way through. A way through to a life far greater than I could have ever imagined possible for myself. You see, the pain changed me, and *how* it changed me was really up to me.

The healing process has so far gone on my entire adult life. It's taken me this long to heal from what was inflicted on me as a child. But, in my healing, there have been lessons that I'm not sure how I would have gained any other way. So my pain has been my gift.

Another teacher of mine, writer and speaker Father Richard Rohr, said, 'If we do not transform our pain, we will most assuredly transmit it – usually to those closest to us: our family, our neighbours, our co-workers, and, invariably, the most vulnerable, our children.'

So what we won't transform, we will transmit.

All our unresolved hurt or trauma gets passed on until someone has the courage to say: 'This all stops with me. I will have the courage now to transform my pain.'

Will this be you?

We are a generation of men who are invited to find new ways of healing. We can move beyond where we are, taking full responsibility and ownership of our own transformation. We can become transformers instead of transmitters.

Much of what has happened to you and been done to you wasn't ever your choice and it wasn't your fault. I'll repeat that: **it wasn't your fault**.

But *now* is your time to become a transformer and a healer. One who has the courage to heal his wounds before you do what has been done many times before: continue to transmit your hurt and your trauma to your children.

'Through my own journey I've learnt that my pain has actually been the biggest invitation to heal.'

Then your shit is theirs, and the cycle just continues with more victims in its path, with another generation of traumatised kids trying desperately to navigate through lives of pain.

Showing up begins with you being open to being challenged and being prepared to be wrong about some things. This can be a scary thing for many of us men. It takes humility to take correction on ideas in our life that aren't working, without taking offence. To be challenged requires our vulnerability, because it requires us acknowledging we need help in an area. Too many of us hate asking for help, often because we either weren't helped when we once asked for it, or because receiving help came with strings attached.

Vulnerability can often be mistaken for weakness, but I assure you there is nothing weak about a man who has the courage to own his own baggage, and begin to address a way of living that currently is not only hurting those directly around him but is destroying him from the inside out, too.

I know with absolute certainty that for you to inflict or project pain onto her, you must be in immense pain yourself. I acknowledge that. And I sit with you in that pain.

As they say: 'Hurt people hurt people.' I write this book as a personal invitation to you to own that hurt and learn new ways to heal it, instead of projecting it onto the women we claim to love the most, and then by default our children who watch and see all. I write this because I also believe that healed people do indeed heal people, and my deepest desire is for a new generation of men who are willing to take ownership for their healing, and who, by default, will then heal others around them.

If our children are watching and learning from our actions, this is the default behaviour they will carry on to their partners, and subsequently their children.

'You cannot be what you cannot see.' So if your children never see positive behaviour from the adults in their life, how can they be better for their own children?

This is how the cycle of violence and abuse continues across generations.

This is *intergenerational trauma* being repeated.

LET ME START by telling you I am sincerely sorry that anyone ever hurt you, and I truly believe, as a man who talks to all kinds of men all day long in my barbershop, that I have never met a man who doesn't innately desire a life of wholeness, where he didn't have to live with the parts of him that hurt the most. No one wants to be a bully or a monster, yet countless men I know are described as just that by their own children.

Is this how you would ever want to be remembered?

You are worthy of a life healed, my Brother, because the alternative is one where every single relationship you have will be your new and temporary rehab facility. You will go from woman to woman, attempting to seek answers to the pain you feel, and no one will ever quite be able to 'fix you'. You'll blame her: 'She's just not strong enough' or 'She couldn't handle it' – and this after she's taken yet another hit, emotionally or physically.

And when she's down there, bruised and battered, unable to give us everything she once did, many of us are quick to dismiss her and move on to another brighter, shinier woman who isn't quite as 'damaged'. And the whole process, or cycle, begins again.

I've heard *all* the excuses:
She just doesn't ever listen to me.
She pushes me to this point.
If only she'd shut up and stop talking at me.
She doesn't give me the respect I deserve.
And when I hear all these things, what I really hear is:
I hate not feeling heard.
This reminds me of a time I felt powerless.
I've never really been part of the conversation.
I haven't felt really loved, so respect is an easier alternative to demand.

RECENTLY, I WAS TALKING to a client whose hair I have been cutting for over seven years. I've seen him at his absolute worst, and at one point about five years ago he missed his regular appointment with me, only for me to find out he had been arrested (again) and was back in prison for a number of reasons. He had been placed in solitary confinement, and I visited him in jail because, in all honesty, I missed him and our conversations, which is what happens when a client becomes a friend and Brother.

I recall vividly how he seemed to me that day; the mask of bravado had come down enough for me to see the real him. A boy whose Father had never shown up and claimed him, as any Father should. A boy whose Mother was so tired of struggling to simply survive, she preferred numbing herself to the point where her drug addiction eventually killed her. It was soon left to the streets to raise him, and raise him they did. Crime, violence and gangs all became part of his adolescent years, along with multiple dysfunctional relationships, where violence and infidelity were the norm.

After he was last released from prison he started to really look at changing his life. I knew he was tired of a life that took more than it ever gave. He started his own business and married his long-time partner. Here was a woman who had stood by him over the years while he had been in and out of prison. Here was a woman who has endured physical violence by his hands. Here was a woman who he called his 'ride-or-die girl' - the kind who stays for better and, more frequently, through worse.

They had their first baby together, and during her pregnancy they started arguing more. He started coming home less, partying more, and eventually started seeing another, much younger woman.

'Throughout this book I want to speak to "him" and call him forward. Because he is who you really are, Brother. He is me. He is us.'

When I asked him about this, genuinely concerned why his life was going back down a path he knew led nowhere, he blamed it all on the arguments. He said they argued because she wanted him to actively seek help for his 'problems', but he thought he had already done the work and changed his life enough. I mean, what more did she want?

I get that. I understand that it's exhausting doing self-work, because I have found myself that it never seems to end. No sooner do you think you are on top of things and you are 'sorted' than something else pops up. I'm always bracing myself for the next lesson that will come along - usually at the most inopportune time. I also give my guy credit where credit is due; because the man who first sat in my barber's chair and the man he is today are seriously worlds apart.

Truthfully, he *had* done some work, and in his mind he had done enough - or as much as he felt he could do.

Here's the thing, though, men: as long as you are living and breathing you'll never be a finished product, so don't stop seeking to better yourself. All of the days of our lives are about growth, and the refinement and evolution of our character. This is because there are different levels of learning. Similar to a school system, you complete a level or grade and graduate that year, only to move up to another, harder grade. And, just like school, if you fail that year you have to repeat it again.

'We're in this together, and if you have ever felt alone in your pain, then this is where I'm here to gently remind you of the truth – that you are far from alone.'

If you find yourself going around and around in life, repeatedly taking the same lessons, then you have to ask yourself what you aren't getting from the lessons that you need to grasp in order to move up to the next level. And once you accept that none of us will ever be a 'finished product' or have it 'all together', as we are all a constant work in progress, it's easier for us to accept that there will always be lessons, and room to grow, so we truly can continually learn at our own pace. Learning is not to be feared, because **all learning is growth**.

So when our women are hitting us up about changing, instead of getting on the defensive, and putting our backs up or making excuses, we have to stand down from our ego, and try to see her intention and motivation. Consider where she is coming from. Consider that she knows you better than other people do. Who we are when we are at home with her is who we really are, more than in any other space we are in.

When we don't take responsibility for our own healing, by

default we put the burden on her, which is exhausting. We collectively need to own that, and realise that if it's that hard for us to change and to rehabilitate ourselves, then it's sure as heck so much harder for her or anyone else to attempt to do it for us.

You can dump, project and transmit your pain onto her all you want, but there is absolutely nothing she can do better for you than what you can do for yourself by owning it.

Often she will try anyway, at the cost of herself, because she so genuinely desires to save you from yourself. I've seen this happen more times than I can count, and the outcome is pretty inevitable. If she rescues you once, then there is a high possibility she will rescue you again, repeatedly, for the full lifespan of what I would call an unhealthy co-dependent relationship. This is because you are both relying on each other playing the rescuer/rescued roles for fulfilment, which is not a healthy relationship dynamic. At the start it can feel really good: she feels needed by you, and you feel looked after by her, which can be nice if you haven't been adequately cared for before. But it ultimately doesn't get either of you anywhere, because neither of you is taking responsibility for yourself.

This was the story I saw repeatedly in my childhood, when the violence got bad enough that the police would come, and Dad would be put in the cells overnight. But as sure as the morning would come, Mum would be there the next day to pick him up and back home he'd be. This was our story. The one where our Mother rescued our Father from any and all real consequences, an unlimited number of times. He'd trash the house in another violent outburst, and she'd clean it up with a bruised face.

So he never learnt. But we, their children, learnt something: that there really were no limits to how far my Mother would go to try to save my Father from himself, even at the expense of herself. And us. What maybe we didn't fully appreciate until we were older, though, was the extent to which our Mother did all of these things to protect us, to take his focus off us. Unfortunately, though, her good intentions had unintended consequences.

As I grew up, I started to understand that by doing all that for him, instead of letting him learn for himself, she unwittingly stunted his learning and healing process dramatically. Her constant attempts to fix what was so broken within him rescued him from the logical consequences of any of his negative behaviour, which meant for us that he continued down the same path for our entire childhoods. This, too, kept him emotionally immature and dependent on her, and she eventually became resentful and tired of having to be this for him. His rehab.

SO WHILE SHE CAN'T ever be your rehab, I want to tell you about the possibility of just what a woman can be for you. Simply put, my wife, Sarah, is my home. With her, I am safe to rehabilitate myself. To have the space and shelter needed to work on and own the shit in my life. When life knocks me down and gives me a lesson that honestly feels like I'm stuck in the middle of the Pacific Ocean drowning, it's her swimming right next to me, telling me to keep my head up. It's her telling me to breathe, and that there is land ahead, so just keep going. She is a voice of encouragement. But she never attempts to swim for both of us, because then we'd both end up drowning.

She is not my rehab, and she will never be, because I don't want to live in a rehab centre! But I do want to live somewhere safe that I can call home, and my home is Sarah.

How has she created this beautiful and safe home?

Good mental health is her priority; she doesn't take on the responsibility of things I am responsible for, like my healing. Boundaries are set so we know where each of us begins and ends. She doesn't rescue me from the consequences of poor decisions I have chosen to make, but she will sit and cry with me when the outcome is painful. She is loyal to the truth, always above comfort. Her speaking truth kindly for me is like someone cleaning out an infected open wound. You have to get the poison out in order for it to heal properly, and give the wound a wipe with disinfectant to kill any bacteria. This stings initially, but it speeds up the healing process hugely. Truth, from her, has shattered old delusions that I didn't even know I lived by. Things taught to me in childhood that I've believed all these years, only because I didn't know, or hadn't seen, better.

She does all this to support me. But she does not take over for me.

My wife is her own person. She doesn't seek my permission or approval, and while I'm grateful she chose me, and chooses me daily, and desires me, she doesn't actually need me. There is something so attractive and wonderful about a woman who doesn't *need* you, but still really *wants* you. More than this, her being so completely herself, in her unique quirkiness, has given me permission to let down my walls and be myself with her.

'Vulnerability can often be mistaken for weakness, but I assure you there is nothing weak about a man who has the courage to own his own baggage, and begin to address a way of living that currently is not only hurting those directly around him but is destroying him from the inside out, too.'

Her example of actively being her own person, while remaining at my side, has given me the confidence to empower myself; to be seen and known, and therefore loved as I really am. For that I am so grateful and blessed.

But she is not my rehab; no woman (or man) ever should be. We can stand in our own mana, and empower ourselves.

EVERY GOOD BARBER HAS the latest tools of the trade that we invest our hard-earned cash in and take good care of, to ensure we can give our clients the best cuts we can. Throughout this book, I'll offer you some tools to try, or ideas to research, that can be helpful in your own healing journey. Tools that can help you to take the best care of yourself that you can.

I believe it all starts with **showing up for yourself**. How do you really start to show up for yourself and become your own advocate and cheerleader?

- Start with sitting down somewhere quiet, and think about who your inner little boy is. For example, Little Matt was a scared, quiet child who didn't want to be bullied or humiliated. He was creative and spent heaps of time alone drawing because it seemed safer than interacting with those around him. Because of this Little Matt was seen as quiet and weak, and became a victim of being bullied and abused by multiple people. This made Little Matt too scared to trust anyone.

- Start writing the first thoughts and ideas that come to you, so you can go over them and see what picture emerges.

- Begin talking to that little boy inside of you. He's still there waiting to be seen and heard. How is he feeling? If you've never seen or heard him, then realise he's the same little boy who is scared and hurt from the trauma you experienced in your childhood.

- Tell him that you love him, and that you are there for him now.

- Treat that little boy with the kindness that you have always wanted. You can do this out loud, or inside your head, but make sure that the words you use are kind and encouraging. It feels weird to start with, but it also helps you to connect with the little boy inside of you who has never been seen.

- Think about your internal dialogue with yourself, or

your 'felt' talk. Are you always telling yourself how stupid you are? That you're dumb, or useless, or a failure? Is that what you were told by other people when you were growing up? Stop doing that right now.

- Use positive affirmations and kind words to speak to your inner child – and doing this regularly will help rewire that brain of yours to think, and act, more kindly towards yourself. As soon as they could talk, my wife and I have taught our children to affirm themselves daily. They have four main affirmations – I am smart, I am kind, I am brave, I am loved – and then they add on their own. You can start with saying these four, and then adding to your own list, too.

- Life is better when you work from the belief that **everyone is doing the best that they can**. Tell yourself that you are doing your best, as are those around you, and follow through on any promises you make to yourself and others. This is the biggest way we learn that we can be trusted, and that we can depend on ourselves to follow through. It can be as simple as promising yourself a walk on the beach, and following through with it, instead of putting it off for another day.

Chapter two

She is not your mother

I MADE A FOOLISH MISTAKE once, when, in a heated argument with my wife, I blurted out: 'You are exactly like my mother!'

I can't remember how the fight even started, or what it was about – but, in all honesty, with us it tends to be over the smallest things. Trust me when I say that my wife and I – we can go from zero to 100 in two seconds flat!

In the early days an argument could start with a harmless conversation about which way to walk to the park, but would end up with me forcibly trying to prove that the way I wanted to go was much quicker, and with her resolutely focused on the way she had already decided to go. The outcome? We ended up stuck in a stalemate, literally going nowhere.

How often do you feel like you're in a stalemate with your partner or wife? Neither of you wanting to budge an inch, so you both effectively remain stuck.

And what I remember about that day when I said those words to Sarah was that I was feeling an old familiar feeling of being unheard rise up. Believing she wasn't hearing me, I felt frustration quickly take over my entire body with an intensity that made my hands shake and my face heat up.

And let's just say that her instant and furious response made it crystal-clear that it wasn't an accusation she wanted to hear . . . ever. I have never repeated it, and I don't think I'll ever be stupid enough to say those words again.

But why did I say them in the first place? What was behind my anger? Those words had come out because whatever we were arguing about - her not agreeing with me and my point - meant that, in my mind, she just wasn't listening to me. Because surely if she *was* listening, she would agree with me, right?

That's an insight I've had to learn over the years: that **someone can, in fact, hear you but not agree with you**. This concept was completely foreign in my childhood, as my experience was that our Father was always to be agreed with and obeyed. If our Mother argued or fought back, then it would always end in violence. This taught me that if she had only just kept the peace, kept her mouth shut, and agreed with whatever he said by not arguing with him, then surely it would be better for all of us, right? We'd have a happier home and less violence if Mum could just do this.

So this was the subconscious belief I took into my marriage: that to disagree was dangerous, and something to be avoided at all costs because it always ended up with violence. The subconscious beliefs within us - the beliefs we often don't even know we have - are the most dangerous ones, because they haven't yet been challenged. Not everything we believe is actually true, and we shouldn't be scared to challenge our own thoughts if we realise they aren't playing out very well in our actual life.

Example: My subconscious belief of 'Being heard means she *must* agree with me' was not working out well for us when disagreements arose. Sarah wasn't prepared to always agree with me, and this meant that I told myself (and truly believed!) that she wasn't hearing me.

This disconnect was a recipe for endless conflict, one that had started in my childhood, watching it play out with my parents. Watching my Mother eventually lose her voice, her opinion and herself. But that's what women did to keep the peace, right? Women should defer to men: this is what my parents' marriage modelled to me. Never mind that this unfair expectation was damaging for both of them.

In my experience watching my parents, less talking equated to less violence. This meant, instinctively, I put ownership on my Mother to control my Father's violence. Even though I knew it was horrible for her living with a man who was so volatile that he lived on a trigger-wire, ready to react to everything and anything. So, in truth, even her silence wasn't safe.

'Sometimes, in a heart-to-heart conversation with a man in my barber chair I might challenge him gently on something he believes with a simple question like: "What is it about that that is so threatening to you?" or: "How's that been working for you so far?"'

Our Mothers are typically our first interaction with a woman. Everything about that interaction shapes us, and our future views of women and how we interact with them. And critically, this includes how we see our Fathers and other men treating them. For me, my most distinctive memories of my Mother are of her always being powerless and in survival mode.

There were countless nights where her screams awoke me and my siblings, as she took yet another beating from our drunk Father. There were the nights when it got too bad even for her to handle, or the neighbours had called the police because of the noise, and then she would bundle us up, to go and stay at a women's refuge shelter for the night.

Even so, it got to the point where it was more disruptive to leave, as we all knew that, without fail, we'd just be back home the next day. So we'd prefer to stay at home, and somehow attempt to just block out the violence happening around us. Eventually the noise of it was a soundtrack we grew so used to hearing that it became easier to live with. It seemed preferable to tough it out than pack up and stay somewhere strange and unfamiliar for the night. As I grew older, at about 13, I got my first pair of headphones, so they gave me a way of blocking out my world while I walked around my neighbourhood listening to my favourite music.

Looking back, I can see that not only had we normalised domestic violence, in the end this was to such a degree that we had become desensitised to it. For example, during my childhood I recall watching the infamous New Zealand movie *Once Were Warriors*. This nineties film is the story of an urban Māori family based in South Auckland, and their struggles with poverty, alcoholism and domestic violence at the hands of the Father, Jake the Muss. I remember watching the beating Jake gave his wife Beth and laughing with my brothers. We laughed because, as kids, we seriously thought the movie was a comedy, and that Beth's hiding was nothing compared with what our Mother received regularly from our Father. I don't think I understood for many years what that did to our thinking as children, but I knew I always thought my Mother was strong to survive what she endured at the hands of our Father.

Decades later, just how these experiences had affected us came out when one of my brothers was arguing with his partner. When she told him how unhappy she was with his behaviour, he angrily responded: 'Harden up! You don't know how lucky you are - you don't have to put up with anything that my Mother survived, so be fucking grateful!'

And there it was.

Subconsciously, us siblings had equated our Mother's survival of extreme abuse with her strength as a woman. We had seen first-hand what she had endured from our Father. But somehow we'd processed it back-to-front: we had made it all about our Mother's strength, her ability to endure. Only much later did I realise our focus should have been the wrongness of her even being put in that situation, on the unconscionable behaviour and violence of our Father. She shouldn't have needed to be making the choices she was making - for us kids as much as for herself. And this warped thinking meant that when it came to having our own relationships with partners in subsequent years, we assumed there really were no limits to what our women should – and could – put up with. Which means that some of the women we have dated have not been treated as they deserved.

If I had stayed in that state of unawareness, and had refused to learn better tools to implement change in my own marriage, I can assure you my wife would not still be with me. And deep down I knew for damn sure that, even though my Mother had put up with years of abuse and projected pain from my Father, Sarah would never allow me to hold our family hostage to such bullshit. She is most definitely *not* my Mother. But, again, the focus should be on my behaviour, not her response to it.

Even so, I knew what her response would have been, because, before we even dated, we were strictly good friends for four years. Our friendship was the time when we both really saw the other. Some consider love to be blind, and in that regard I would say genuine platonic friendship is actually very illuminating, because with no one trying to impress the other, you can see someone for who they are.

We had met when she was an event manager for a non-profit aid and development agency, and I was a member of a local hip-hop band that she had toured as part of a campaign she was managing. I had seen first-hand the kind of woman she was before we ever entered into any kind of romantic relationship. One thing I admired about her – other than what a devoted single Mother she was to her young daughter, and loving guardian of her younger teenage sister – was her love of self-progress, and taking her own mental health and healing seriously. She wasn't content to just sit there and wait for anyone else to rescue her. She was always truthful and had insightful things to share, so conversations with her were stimulating and enjoyable, and led me to checking out my own thought processes on numerous occasions.

Sarah is of mixed heritage (Māori and New Zealand-born European), and I'm a New Zealand-born Sāmoan, and although we could be mistaken for being worlds apart or physical polar opposites, we both have our own individual stories of childhood trauma and extreme pain and abandonment.

Very easily we could project or transfer that pain onto each other. And in the beginning stages of our relationship we did! We had moments when our individual 'hurts' from past experiences conflicted with the other's equally painful 'hurts'.

For example, I hate feeling cornered and interrogated with a million questions in times of conflict, because this reminds me of the times I felt accused and blamed or punished wrongly for things I hadn't done as a child. In such moments I'd feel overwhelmed with what was coming at me and I wouldn't be able to think properly, so I would start reacting, and saying things in the heat of the moment that weren't how I truly felt. It's the classic psychological reaction that occurs in response to a perceived attack or threat - we choose either fight or flight. To stand our ground and stand up for ourselves - and hopefully defeat the enemy or threat - or run away and protect ourselves. And when it got like this between us, I'd usually prefer to leave the argument, to go away, calm down, and get my thoughts together.

My wife, on the other hand, hates it if dialogue stops in moments of conflict, because she wants answers to make sense of what is happening. Her questions are her way of seeking clarity and awareness. She isn't trying to attack and overwhelm me, but to sort out our differences and find a resolution. If I leave the argument before this occurs, she feels abandoned, or that she isn't a priority. This triggers in her the deep feelings of rejection she had in her childhood, from being abandoned by her significant people when she needed them.

So together we have committed to always prioritising growth over comfort, no matter how hard it gets, and being open and honest no matter the cost. Even in the hard times. By doing this, we come together and grow in understanding over our arguments - we dissect them after the heat of the moment, and take from that moment of fire the gem the heat has forged.

In this way our arguments and disagreements have been key to realising what triggers each of us, and then have guided us in doing some self-work in our own therapy sessions or time.

There is no monastery like a marriage: a space where you're

almost forced into consistent self-examination, reflection and refinement. The people closest to you are the ones who highlight what needs work and therefore raise the question: **are you willing to do that work?**

Keep that picture in your mind the next time you feel or hear yourself overreacting to something said to you in innocence by your partner. Ask yourself what is really triggering you to react this way. What's 'sore in you' that requires some attention and healing? And when did you first feel that hurt? This is where I believe we all begin in our healing journey.

My childhood home is where it all began for me. That three-bedroom state house that housed me, my three older half-sisters and my four brothers.

Our parents spoke little English, so life for us was going to school and speaking English and being a New Zealander, but coming home and being Sāmoan, being spoken to by our parents only in Sāmoan. Growing up Polynesian, you are taught that respect of elders and your parents is paramount. As a Polynesian child you are not to ever dare question them or their authority on anything. Asking questions was not an acceptable part of our childhood, no matter how confusing and dysfunctional life was.

Because my Mother was so busy surviving vicious attacks from my drunk Father, she turned to gambling for solace, which in turn led to compulsive lying (especially when it came to money). For this reason I grew up with a very warped idea of what women's characters were like, and for most of my twenties I subconsciously believed women, on the whole, to be very untrustworthy.

It is these subconscious perceptions we acquire through our experiences as children that we need to be fully aware of as adults, so that we can challenge them and test their truth before projecting them onto our partners.

Sometimes, in a heart-to-heart conversation with a man in my barber chair, I might challenge him gently on something he believes with a simple question like: 'What is it about that that is so threatening to you?' or: 'How's that been working for you so far?'

It's crucial to continually challenge our subconscious thinking.

He won't always have an answer for me right then, but a good question can provoke a fresh perspective, and sometimes trigger him to make changes.

It's not acceptable to keep unhealthy thinking or toxic beliefs going in your life just because you've 'always had them' or 'that's how it goes in our family'. For the sake of our children, it's up to us to say: 'This is where the bullshit stops!'

To do this, we need to look clearly at what is in front of us, and not let what lies behind us distort our view. For example, my own wife is clearly trustworthy, with a high standard of integrity, but even so, initially I was wary. Is anyone really trustworthy? I wondered.

My questioning was because I could not simply accept the evidence in front of me, but felt the need to evaluate it - and protect myself - by referring to my past. And in my past experience those closest to me were not trustworthy. In fact, they had proved themselves to be the least trustworthy: it was those who were closest to me, including my own parents and other relatives, who had physically, mentally and sexually abused me.

To say that I believed 'trusting people is dangerous' is an understatement.

For those of us who have been hurt and harmed, many of us struggle to trust others. Sure, we need to acknowledge our past, and what those experiences have taught us, but we also need to accept that life does not always - and need not - repeat itself. To do this we need to have the courage to look at the present on its own terms, to trust the evidence that is before our eyes now. It is a matter of balancing the lessons of the past with being open to new possibilities. My advice is to build such trust in increments. People should not be dismissed before they are given an opportunity to show who they are. But nor should anyone be trusted in all things immediately. Too many people give out almost everything to a new partner straight away, only to be incredibly disappointed when their trust is shattered.

Whether giving people trust in all areas too quickly, or not trusting people at all, neither option gives us what we want.

So trust is incremental. There is give and there is take, and with time it grows. Here's how I slowly began to trust Sarah when, initially, I did not believe women to be trustworthy. When we were just friends, I would tell her something that was hard for me to share, and then I'd judge her reaction and see if she would tell anyone else. When she proved herself there, I would try another area.

It's alarming to me how quickly people move in together, especially when there are children involved. It takes time for someone to prove himself or herself trustworthy. I learnt over time, by her consistent actions, that Sarah could be trusted, and that she kept her word, not over-promising, not under-delivering. This was hugely important to me, because trust had never been modelled well throughout my childhood.

'For those of us who have been hurt and harmed, many of us struggle to trust others. Sure, we need to acknowledge our past, and what those experiences have taught us, but we also need to accept that life does not always – and need not – repeat itself.'

Effective communication was also something that was never modelled to me, growing up. In the early days of my relationship with Sarah, there were times when I would feel extremely disappointed that she hadn't shown up for me in exactly the way I wanted her to. It wasn't that she hadn't wanted to be there for me, she just hadn't realised that I wanted her to do something in a particular way. And because I hadn't communicated what I wanted to her, she had no idea. How could she? Yet I would react badly because I was so disappointed. She would then have to sort through my reactions to identify the real issue, and then explain to me that she'd had no idea what I'd wanted her to do. Another time, all I had to do was communicate clearly with her what I needed, and if she could be there for me, she absolutely would.

And this perhaps is another example of learning to work with what is in front of you: your partner is not a mind-reader. Some of us are so scared of being rejected or abandoned that we don't communicate our needs clearly to those we love, effectively expecting them to be mind-readers. When they fail to read our minds, and disappoint us, the hurt we feel is magnified; it reminds us of a much deeper pain that has existed since we were neglected or abandoned as children. And again we find ourselves turning away from the here and now, and emotionally reaching back and responding to the past. But it's unfair and unrealistic to project those hurts onto our wife or partner. They can't be expected to show up for all those other people who didn't show up for us in the past. These days, I'm more mindful of identifying and clearly communicating my needs with Sarah, instead of expecting her to read my mind and fix my problems. The focus is on us, here and now, acting; not on others, in the past, reacting.

GROWING UP AS A Sāmoan boy also meant that our Mother did most, if not all, of the family domestic tasks or chores. I have never seen my Father clean at all, and my Mother did the majority of the cooking. Occasionally my Father would cook, but it was always strictly for himself. He would make a small pot of something – enough for himself to eat – but never for our Mother, or us kids. His role, as he saw it, was to go to work to earn money, and that was it. The housework was not something he invested in at all, even though my Mother also worked over the years to bring in money.

When my older half-sisters eventually came to live with us at different times, it was expected that they would also undertake the domestic tasks, as well as serve and look after us, their younger brothers. Looking back, they probably weren't thrilled about this. Culturally, it was just a given in our family, so this also set up my thinking – expecting women to serve their men with domestic duties.

I think what we have to remember is that, while our wife or partner is a Mother, she is not *our* Mother. Our role, as her partner, is to equally and positively contribute to our relationship, and to our family dynamic. You are not one of her children, and it's unfair for her to be put in the position of having to constantly ask you for your help, like you're doing her a favour. She is not your Mother, and she is also not your babysitter or caregiver.

Sarah was the first woman I ever lived with in a relationship. She made it clear very early on after we moved in together that I would need to pull my weight around the house. I must admit we had some very heated discussions on what life would look like, and my expectations of her. She pointed out that while I did go to work at the barbershop, she also worked on our business from home, along with doing all the cooking, washing and cleaning. She is house-proud and enjoys cooking, but she said that, while she was happy to do those tasks, this didn't mean she should be treated like a doormat, or have the expectation placed on her that it was her 'duty'. At this stage we had only our elder daughter, and Sarah had been a single Mother to her for over 10 years, so she already ran a pretty tight ship.

I agreed that I was happy to contribute, and I certainly didn't want my living with them to feel like more work for her, so she assigned me a night a week to cook, and a few specific tasks to do around the house weekly. I can tell you proudly that I now clean the bathroom better than anyone, even if it takes a full bottle of bleach and a few hours!

I learned more about the load women carry when Sarah was pregnant with our son - my first biological child. She was extremely sick the entire time, always vomiting, and had an alarming tendency to bleed a lot. She worked from home on our business, and we were opening a new barbershop at the time, so there was a lot to do. Suddenly she didn't want to cook, as it made her so nauseous, and she couldn't do much around the house either.

Once you have children together, the dynamic changes. You, and what you require, are not the sole focus of her world anymore, as she only has so much energy to give out daily, and suddenly all the things she may have allowed in your relationship pre-children might not be so doable for her now. I hear so many men complain about this, but in reality I think it's a small price to pay for the gift they give us of Fatherhood.

Many of us have grown up watching our Mothers do everything, and had Fathers who did very little to support them at home. This was what I witnessed first-hand growing up. One particularly vivid memory I have is of my Mother when she was pregnant with my youngest brother. I was about eight years old. As we grew up with no washing machine, I remember her on her knees hunched over the bathtub, heavily pregnant and crying. She was talking to herself out loud, saying that this was not the life her Father had wanted for her.

She had received yet another hiding, but there she was, still washing our clothes in her condition. We were never really allowed in there with her – she always kicked us out if we went in there while she was doing the washing – but I would sometimes watch her from the hallway, seeing her put all the clothes in the bath, and then bending over them with a bar of soap and scrubbing them by hand. Then she would wring all of the clothes out until her hands were red, and hang them outside. It was an arduous task, especially given the quantity of dirty clothing my siblings and I produced!

I have another vivid image of my Mother, sitting by the dining room window, looking outside when my Father was at work. Her eyes were so sad. I remember asking her if she was alright, and her response would always be: 'I'm OK, Son.' I didn't know how to help her as a child, but I thought to myself: 'I wish I could make her eyes happy.'

Her sad eyes have been imprinted on my soul and have been with me my entire life.

This was Christchurch, New Zealand, in 1994. This was us living in a three-bedroom government house, with between five and eight children (depending on whether my sisters were there) and sometimes extra relatives. It doesn't seem that long ago. Yet we live in a completely different cultural climate now. Women now lead vastly different lives from the generations of women before them. Education, and more career choices, mean that women have infinitely more options available to them than they ever had in previous times. And arguably more state and social support if they need to remove themselves and their children from a bad situation.

So, while it was normal in my childhood to never see our Father lift a finger to help our Mother, I refuse this to ever be a norm in my home. I have seen incredible women around me blossom into motherhood with a strength that surpasses everything else. Watching Sarah nurture our babies is by far one of the most beautiful sights I have been privileged to witness. Watching sisters of mine being free to give out more than our Mother was ever able to encourages me as a Father that it's possible to heal the trauma we've experienced, to be more for our children than what we had.

My Mother endured terrible things for us kids, and at an unfathomable cost to herself. She was confronted not only by my Father's unremitting, desensitising, normalised violence but by an extended family, neighbourhood and church community that again and again turned a blind eye to her suffering. With no money, she toughed it out, and did the best she could for us. Held back by cultural expectations of duty, and with little education and poor English, she could not access the social support that might have allowed us to escape.

Looking back, perhaps that endurance is the expression of love that she could not always voice to us. And perhaps the unforgettable image I have of her hunched over the bathtub washing our endless piles of laundry is why my own preferred language of love is service?

But I now live in a completely different world.

My beloved is not my Mother, but she is the Mother of my children, and that has gifted me with Fatherhood - my greatest role, and the greatest opportunity of my life to heal. Fatherhood is my chance to show up daily, in the small tasks and the big moments. These are the memories my own children are filing away in their subconscious. **What am I teaching them?**

Consider the following...

- Think about some of the subconscious thoughts and beliefs you hold onto. What are they? Where did they come from? How are they working out for you in your daily life?

- What are your perceptions of women, and of families? Where did these ideas come from? Have you changed them over time?

- Think about some of the things that trigger you. These are the things (words, moments, actions) that will make you instantly react – like someone has stuck a hot poker into you. What makes you instantly react?

- What tools and strategies do you have if someone triggers you? How do you deal with these feelings?

- How do you deal with sharing work in and around the home? Do you deliberately do a bad job so your wife or partner doesn't ask you to help again? Do you take over everything, or expect things to be done in a particular way, as if your way is the only way?

- What do you do when you don't feel heard? How do you react?

- How do you identify and clearly communicate what you need to others?

Chapter three

She is not your absent father

WHEN I FINISH AT THE BARBERSHOP for the day and arrive home, it is a joyous reunion. My children all excitedly rush to me the moment I get in. 'Daddy!' they scream, as they fight with each other for my exclusive attention.

There is always this little happy/sad feeling in my heart. Happy because, like many children, my precious darlings know they are loved and safe with me, their Father. But sad, because this was not my childhood experience at all. I was always wondering how not to make my Father angry. I wondered what would trigger him next. It was almost a game to think ahead to remove or stop anything that might set him off.

As I grew older, I realised there was actually nothing I could do to predict his unpredictable behaviour because he was so erratic. I simply tried my best to avoid him, as much as I possibly could, while still living in the same house. In that way I defensively detached from him before I hit puberty. This means that I kept all interaction to an absolute minimum. I'd only engage with him if not engaging with him meant I'd get a hiding.

When I think back, I knew things were bad when the physical beatings were so much more preferable to the emotional beatings we would take from him. The belittling words or the barrage of humiliation he would inflict on us for his own amusement. He would say the cruellest things constantly: 'You're useless' or 'You're a good-for-nothing', or refer to us as 'dickheads' and 'shit'. The worst thing he would say to us was in Sāmoan, and translated means 'I curse you', but worse than that, it means 'I curse your life and you don't have my blessing', which I suppose is something most of us Polynesian children aspire to obtain. It cuts deep to hear your Father tell you this regularly. Those words never go away; they still ring around your mind long after the bruises fade.

My Father was physically absent through periods of our life, too. He was in jail for an extended period when my two older brothers were young, and then he would regularly be locked up in the cells, or do short stints for months at a time in Christchurch Men's Prison. This was on those rare occasions when he would actually be charged with domestic violence. Usually he got away with all the beatings he gave my Mother.

We would regularly go with my Mother to visit him in prison while he was inside, and he was always there behind the glass, crying and apologising to us. But from a young age I knew that he was only sorry because he was feeling the consequences of actions that would usually go unpunished, and because he was sober while in jail. These were the only periods of time he was consistently sober. I do not recall him ever hitting my Mother on the rare, brief occasions he was sober on the outside. But, immediately, the moment he was back out, the drinking and the violence would return, almost as if he had never been away.

He never took these times off the bottle as an opportunity to look deep within himself, to see what it was he was actually trying to self-medicate away. I believe his behaviours went way beyond the expression of cultural and social 'norms' of the time. It was intergenerational. He, too, was ferociously protecting a damaged little boy within, but, for whatever reason, he never allowed that little boy to be seen and healed and liberated.

Perhaps it is that little boy I now occasionally glimpse when I see my Father being a Grandfather to my children?

There was also the period of time when he left us for several years to move cities and be with another woman. To be honest, I didn't miss him at all. Life was far less stressful with him not there, and we all felt the freedom his absence gifted us. His presence robbed us of the freedom you should feel as a child, because I never felt free when there was always someone to fear, and something to worry about. Always having to be hyper-aware of your surroundings and potential threats, always ready to get out of a situation if you could.

'I have learnt in my job as a barber that family violence and childhood trauma do not discriminate by colour, or by wealth.'

The day my Father unexpectedly returned when I was 13 years old is forever etched on my mind. He gave me a hiding outside on the driveway for not opening the garage door for him. I knew what that hiding was, too. It was a reminder of who he was, and his position in our home, whether he came or went. It was a reminder that he was to be feared and his authority never challenged.

When I use the term 'absent Father' I am referring to a man who is absent in his role as a Father to the child he has brought into this world. Make no mistake: you can have an absent Father who lives with you every day of your childhood. Abusive fathering is also absent fathering, as you are simply not fully present in giving your children what they need from you. There is nothing present about a man who is living in his past pain and trauma so deeply that he is now inflicting it on his own children.

If you are not present, then you are, indeed, absent.

By the time I was a teenage boy, I was completely shut down and suicidal. I didn't trust anyone and couldn't be in a close, real relationship with any adults - especially older males in a position of authority in my life. I would lie to protect myself, and I had plenty of masks to hide behind. All because I had never been adequately nurtured in a safe environment, which meant that genuine connection with other people - and men in particular - felt impossible.

They say that every boy measures his masculinity at the deepest level against his Father. My masculinity had taken a beating, and who could I connect with in my world to find the answers that I desperately needed?

Not with my own Father, clearly.

Not with the priest either. My teacher at the Catholic school was the first to sexually abuse me and a male cousin while we were both altar boys.

Not even with my close uncle who had seen the childhood I had suffered, but who still manipulated our relationship to eventually rape me at 13 years of age.

I lacked a safe connection with any males older than I was who I could trust; by then, I trusted no one. When you are in pain like I was, your natural reaction is to stay behind one of your many masks and pretend. You tell everyone you are 'all good' and 'I've got this', and for years I would put on a mask and hide my pain.

To hide my pain I was very introverted and appeared shy, with little to offer anyone. I hid in my music and art and video games. Always listening to something or watching something or drawing - anything to block out my shit reality. Escapism via creativity saved me in many ways, and I hid from anyone seeking any kind of relationship with depth. I was terrified at being really seen by others.

But deep down I knew I had to find someone to help me, and I had to be real with my pain before I choked on the words I was biting back daily. I had to dig deep to find the courage to slowly remove my mask and connect heart-to-heart with another person, to say: **'This is who I am, and I need help!'**

TO DO THIS REQUIRES A SCARY THING called vulnerability.

My 'white Mama' Brené Brown (yes, we even have the same last name, so I have officially adopted her!) taught me more about this topic than anyone else, and I invite you to look her up and watch her TED talk, *The Power of Vulnerability*. Brené trained as a social worker, and she has researched shame and vulnerability for many years.

Those two words – shame and vulnerability – are inextricably linked. The word 'vulnerability' comes from the Latin *vulnus*, which means 'wound', and being vulnerable opens us up to being easily hurt, influenced or attacked. But Brené taught me that vulnerability is *not* weakness. It is taking an emotional risk, and exposing ourselves to uncertainty. Brené says: 'Vulnerability is our most accurate measurement of courage. It is also the birthplace of innovation, creativity, and change.'

Shame is the fear of disconnection, and Brené says it has two big loops: 'I'm never good enough' and 'Who do you think you are?'

Shame is not guilt either. Shame says 'I am bad', while people who feel guilt say 'I did a bad thing'. Brené also says that people who feel shame also may have one or all of the following issues: addiction, depression, bullying, suicidal thoughts and urges, eating disorders, violence and aggression; whereas people who feel guilt usually have none of these issues.

Listening to Brené absolutely transformed how I viewed my own shame, and it encouraged me to step into a more vulnerable existence.

For me, vulnerability first meant asking for help. This was terrifying for me as an abused teenage boy, because I was potentially putting myself in harm's way to (at worst) possibly be abused again, or (at the very least) be let down yet again. But when I did finally reach out to a youth leader and tell him that I needed help, my vulnerability was met with empathy. He took me to Burger King for lunch and really listened to me and to the pain that I shared. I don't recall his words at all, but I recall how he left me feeling: powerful. And our conversation helped me to take back control and leave home at 15.

When I finally had the courage to really be seen, my confidence grew as I discovered not everyone wanted to harm me. First, it was with the youth leader, then slowly other close friends, and finally with my wife. I learnt first-hand that since most of our hurts come through relationships, so too will our healing. But our healing can absolutely *not* come at the expense of another, but rather in collaboration and support of each other.

I have also since realised that a majority of men I have met through my work would wear their own masks of staunch pride and anger, but underneath they were little boys like I once was, who were cut as children and now stand there as adults, bleeding to death all over women and children who never cut them.

There are men like this everywhere – in cities all over the world. We sadly have prisons full of them! We have bloodstained men in suits in high-powered, corporate positions and even wearing uniforms. We have men of all different colours. I have learnt in my job as a barber that family violence and childhood trauma do not discriminate by colour, or by wealth.

Once I awakened to this realisation, I decided that this would be my job for the rest of my life. That I would create a safe place to assist men to take their masks off, one at a time. Barbering and my barbershop have become the vehicle for me to do this. The social media platforms I grew became another vehicle, as did the programmes I now facilitate in prison. All are vehicles for men to feel safe enough to be seen.

I distinctly recall a day in my barbershop in the early days when we were all hard at work. There were six barbers rostered on cutting at the time and we were all fully booked, so there were 12 men in my shop. When you walk in the door of my barbershop, it has a distinctive, masculine smell of wood and patchouli, men's cologne and the sweat of hard-working men. We often have old-school Motown tunes and nineties hip-hop playing. It's alive with masculine energy – noisy and quiet at the same time, with clippers buzzing and conversations going on across the room. Each chair is a quiet space within the noise.

I had just finished a client and was waiting for my next one to arrive. I remember looking around my shop and observing that I knew every single client personally, and, of course, all of my barbers. I realised that every single man cutting or being cut was also a product of an abusive or absent Father. It sent a chill down my spine, as I realised the effects that these Fathers' absence had had on each one of us.

Some of these men had multiple children they weren't raising; others had failed, abusive or dysfunctional relationships. Some had issues with communication, poor mental health, a few couldn't read, some had issues with violence, one had turned to gang life, some had been in and out of prison. One had grooming and hygiene problems as he had never been shown how to clean himself adequately. A few had real issues with conflict, and learning the difference between constructive feedback and criticism from authority, some had very little confidence and deep-rooted insecurity that had come as a result of little to no masculine nurture, and some had learnt to numb away their pain with alcohol and drugs.

It resonated deep within me at that particular point, seeing the effects of what I call a fatherless generation; a high number of men who, in the absence of healing from the atrocities of their abandonment and abuse, were now self-medicating.

And our women and children have become the collateral damage in the process of this.

To turn things around requires dedication and hard work. If you look at an old car that needs restoration, it takes a lot of work. It's the same with working on ourselves: sometimes we need to strip ourselves right back to the bone, and do the work of restoring ourselves, layer by layer, until we are whole again. This restoration project on ourselves needs to be taken seriously if we are ever to move forward from surviving to thriving, to positively impact the generation after us by living healed lives.

The first step in this process is accepting what has happened to you, and realising the enormity of it and how it affects your daily life. Many of us have sometimes had to block out the events that traumatised us as children simply because they were too painful to live through again. I know this because there are things I have no recollection of until I sit down with my siblings and discuss them in rare conversations where we talk about hard things. It's only then that a memory resurfaces and we fill in the blanks for each other. When you reach acceptance, you can begin to grieve for what has been taken from you.

Having said this, the grieving process is different for all of us, and the timing of it varies. In my case, there were many nights alone in my twenties, long before I had a relationship with my wife, where I just gave myself permission to cry. I would sit in my bedroom alone and feel the grief of a lost childhood. I'd feel the pain of having a Father who never showed up for me in the way I needed. I felt anger at his inability to heal himself, and at how that had subsequently affected myself, my siblings and my Mother in varying ways that required us to now heal from the wounds he had inflicted.

'Did I have what it took to father my own son well when I hadn't been properly fathered? This question continually resurfaced.'

It was in those times - through surrendering to my tears - that the deep pain, hurt and betrayal could surface and begin to be felt. These feelings deserve acknowledgement. Many times when I've sat with my own anger I've found it really goes by other names. I guess anger is just a far more acceptable emotion for us men to feel than having to work out if we're actually feeling:

Fear	Not being heard	Humiliation
Frustration	Inadequacy	Grief
Disappointment	Rejection	Sadness
Abandonment	Shame	Trauma

ANOTHER SEASON OF SHEDDING TEARS arrived with the birth of my son. If ever I was sent an invitation to heal, he was it.

From the moment he was born, the weight of my emotions was overwhelming.

Did I have what it took to father my own son well when I hadn't been properly fathered? This question continually resurfaced. And although I often doubted myself, I didn't let this disempower me. Instead, I let it motivate me: I actively sought advice from other, more seasoned Fathers.

Brother, please don't ever be ashamed to ask for assistance in areas you don't have knowledge of and experience in. Every client who ever sat in my chair who was a Father I humbled myself before, and asked advice from. There is no shame in seeking to be better than you are. Our children depend on us to do this. I wanted so badly to be the Father I never had for my son that I just decided I would do the work needed, whatever it took.

I would speak with Fathers at all ages and stages of their Fatherhood journey. I would listen to podcasts and audiobooks on the subject. I would attend parenting workshops and seminars, read articles and manuals, all in the hope that I could learn better than what was given to me, for the sake of my children. It cost me only some time, and it strengthened my willingness to learn. There are plenty of free resources out there, and we have so much more available to us than our Fathers ever did. There are no excuses, my Brother - you, too, can be better than what you were given.

The next step in my journey of healing from the absence of my Father was to physically forgive the man who had abandoned us. This is easier said than done. For while I could say I had already forgiven him, had I really?

After I have shared my story at various speaking events I'm invited to, I am often asked about what has happened to my parents and, more importantly, how things are with my Father.

Today, I consciously choose to see my Father through eyes of compassion. This in no way minimises his behaviour or condones what he did to us. I have chosen to forgive him purely so I can move on from that season of my life with no bitterness. To not forgive him would leave me stuck there, and still a victim of what he did. I knew that instead, for myself, I had to publicly surrender my need to hold him so tightly to those actions from the past.

In saying this, it's important to understand that forgiveness isn't necessarily a one-time event. For me, with some of my abusers it is a daily choice. Part of this is realising that forgiveness is always about you - not them. It's the gift we give ourselves. I choose to forgive so I can sleep at night and have peace with my life. Then I'm in the space to give my children the best of me. But I didn't get to a place of forgiving my Father or any of my abusers overnight. It has taken time and constant surrender to get there. It has cost me. It has cost me my need to hold tight to my version of justice. Some days I might be angry, or in tears, or grieving, but I attempt to make a conscious daily decision from my heart to forgive. This looks like me, in real-time moments, saying **'I forgive you, I forgive you, I forgive you'** to members of my family even when part of me feels they don't deserve my forgiveness.

Some people want vengeance for being hurt, and I understand that, too. You want to release the energy that is still built up inside you, but the reality is the people who hurt you may never get what you define as 'justice'. You may never be able to get your revenge. And even if you hurt them back more than they ever hurt you, this will not remove the pain inside of you. I believe that life will teach those who harm others. Some call it karma - but there's no hiding from it. You don't need to run around trying to punish others - they do that to themselves. I don't hold onto the need for a specific resolution, or any particular outcome.

My only focus is my own heart, my own spirit, and my own energy, as this is what is feeding my children, and they are who my life is purposed for.

Forgiveness isn't dependent on the other person changing. I live in hope they will, but chances are they may not.

And just because you forgive someone, that doesn't mean you need to be in a relationship with them, or forget what they did. I've had to learn the hard reality of forgiving and loving family members from afar. That's where having firm boundaries in place can help.

Often people don't really understand what boundaries are,

so they feel almost abandoned or rejected when you enforce yours. Those who benefited from me having no boundaries in place aren't going to like it when suddenly they don't have an all-access pass to me. Now, in my thirties, I don't have close relationships with those who cannot handle being told 'no', because, in a genuine relationship of reciprocity, each person should be able to say 'no' and have that respected and accepted. When you have boundaries, you can have hard conversations with people you love.

You can say things like:

'I won't let you speak to me like that.'

'I won't let you do that to me.'

'If you behave like that and prove yourself to be untrustworthy, then there are consequences. For example, I won't be doing any kind of joint financial venture with you.'

I'VE LEARNT BRENÉ'S WORDS to be true: 'The most compassionate and generous people are the most boundaried.' It's impossible to fully love another if you have no boundaries, because your relationship will involve endless self-sacrifice. Boundaries exist to demonstrate **this is where I end, and this is where you begin**, and, actually, I get to determine what that looks like. Boundaries also enable you to meet the other person on a middle ground that is comfortable and determined by both of you.

In 2014, at the opening of the barbershop I have now, I chose to cut my Father's hair, as the very first man I officially cut in my shop, and I publicly forgave him, with all my family, barbers and clients as witnesses.

It was not an easy process. It cost me a few of my masks, it cost me my pride, and I would be lying if I said that forgiving him came easily. It didn't. It took years of surrendering my pain behind closed doors to be able to forgive him openly. So you may ask 'Why did you even bother?' It's not like he deserved my forgiveness, right? And to be honest, on that night he came late, drunk, and only because my younger brother Paul forced him into the car and brought him along.

Brother, we have to learn to heal from the things we never got an apology for. It's in this surrender that we become free. In that moment my Father was unaware of what I offered, but I offered it anyway.

I guess, on my journey I learnt to see the man behind the mask of alcoholism and the violence. I see a man who lost his Mother at a young age, and who had not adequately learnt how to express his own emotions. A man who was so completely shut down emotionally that rage was all that seemed acceptable to express the pain he felt on the inside. I see a man who had moved countries with very little, to try to better his situation so that his children could have a better life, and who found it difficult to communicate in a whole new culture that really looked down on him, an immigrant of colour working in a factory.

'Forgiveness is always about you – not them. It's the gift we give ourselves.'

I see that to do what he did to us - his own children and the woman he claimed to love - meant he must have been in such pain himself. When I see that man, he is no longer the monster of my childhood, but a man bound by fear who also needs love and connection, as we all do, to heal and grow.

The barbershop helped me see that man, because every day there are plenty of others like him who sit in my chair. And if I couldn't forgive and love my own father, then I knew I had no business journeying with other men in my city as they attempted to heal. The barbershop helped me become this man, too. Journeying with men, in the way I have done, has helped me to release the un-forgiveness I carried for a long time towards a man who terrorised me for most of my childhood. In releasing this, I am released to be the Father for my children I always desired for myself.

I wholeheartedly live by the concept that we teach people how to love us. And with this in mind I want to invite every single one of you who has struggled with absent parents to grasp the concept of re-parenting yourself. In other words, teach yourself how to love yourself, and actually show up for yourself and give it 100%.

For me, this has been me teaching myself to show up for myself in ways that I need now, and in ways that seem unfamiliar to what I knew as a child.

Brother, it's time for a lesson in parenting ourselves. I've met too many men who struggle to parent their children because they haven't learnt to care for themselves. In my experience, before any men get pushed by the courts into any kind of mandated parenting course, they need to take a course in fathering *themselves*. Those of us who have been abused, neglected, rejected or abandoned by parents often have the ache of a lonely soul that has never been nurtured adequately. We've missed out on vital connections with the people we needed to affirm, support and encourage us while we were at crucial stages of growth. How can anyone give what they haven't received?

This manifests itself with the lonely soul walking through life, trying to cope and self-medicate to seek comfort with a huge variety of survival kits. Things like dependency on alcohol, or food, or substances, or sex. Trying to feel worthy by over-achieving at work, or in sport. Even emotionally isolating away from the real world with things like excessive playing of video games, thus avoiding genuine relationships with real people, because a virtual world seems easier to navigate. Or we become co-dependent on the first soul who shows us any interest and live in a relationship of constant dysfunction.

While the survival kits are as varied as the individual, the results all turn out the same. No survival kit can ever really soothe the longing inside that the absence of a parent feels like.

I've come to understand that I have to be the affirming, encouraging, supportive voice in my own life that I needed growing up. So I practise talking to myself as if I am a small child. Especially in hard moments when I feel like I've failed. 'Matt,' I'll say, 'I'm so proud of you for trying. Maybe you didn't get to where you wanted to with that, but you showed up, and you gave it your best, and look what you learnt in the process!'

The key is to speak really kindly. It's easy for your self-talk to be brutal. It's easy to kick yourself when you are down, and let those old familiar voices tell you that you are useless, and stupid, and will never amount to anything. But to re-parent ourselves, and be the parent now that we once needed, the key is in being kind and patient – really kind. The same kindness I extend to my children now, I've had to learn to extend to myself.

Most of us didn't experience much kindness in our childhoods, but when you experience it finally, after years of having none? I promise that it heals the tender, sore heart like nothing else, because, finally, someone is showing up for you. It just happens that the person showing up is you.

'There is no shame in seeking to be better than you are.'

If your Father was absent, or abusive like mine, you have to learn to give yourself what you need now. You have to stop hoping that he, or some other big person (your boss, or your coach, or your teacher) is going to show up and give you what you need. You can teach yourself how to meet your own emotional and physical needs in small, practical ways. For example, as I said before, if you say you'll do something for yourself, then keep your word and do it. This might be as small as getting up when your alarm first goes off, or finishing a course or educational pursuit you've started. It could look like saying 'No' if you don't want to do something, versus saying 'Yes' and not following through with it, or doing it resentfully. This is all teaching you to show up for yourself, and it is an important part of growing in emotional maturity and capability.

This isn't said to cast blame on my Father either. My Father was absent for us, but he was also absent for himself. He didn't have what I needed, but he also didn't have the right skills to parent himself after losing his Mother so young. I've forgiven him for his lack in parenting me, and I've let go of the need for him to show up for me how I need now.

This has freed me to enjoy who he is now, as my children's Grandfather. As a Father now, I walk my kids around to his house for regular visits. We never stay longer than an hour, sometimes it might be just a 10-minute pop-in - it's a relationship on my terms. The visits are never long enough to escalate into any sort of situation I don't choose to be in. I think it's important for us abused children, as adults, to be able to have a relationship on *our* terms.

'Brother, we have to learn to heal from the things we never got an apology for. It's in this surrender that we become free.'

My parents divorced but still chose to live together until my Mother passed away in December 2020. They said it was 'out of convenience', but I say 'out of companionship', too. My Mother would say 'Better the devil you know than the devil you don't', and while he was no longer physically abusive to her, and hadn't been for years, they had this love/hate relationship where they seemed to drive each other crazy, but then would always end up back with each other.

Dad gives my children treats and laughs at their antics when we visit. He tells funny stories and the children find him hilarious. I wouldn't leave my children alone in his care, but in these fleeting moments my children get to see the good within him - the good I never saw when I was their age. I'm happy for them, and I'm happy for him that he finally gets this.

I've never met a single human who has no good at all inside them. You find what you seek, and in the moments I see him with my children, I see him in childlike innocence, so far removed from the absent Father. He is now the present Grandfather.

In this role I see redemption, and the chance for him to be what he never could be for me.

Chapter four

She is not your shame

HUMILIATION WAS A HUGE PART of how I was disciplined as a child growing up. It was pretty common among many of the Polynesian children of my generation. It wasn't always enough to be physically beaten by my parents, because after a while my brothers and I became desensitised to the violence. The pain threshold of what we could physically endure also seemed to increase, so the beatings just didn't have the same desired effect.

It's like my parents knew this, and so, to keep us subdued and submitted to their authority, they would have to find other ways to break us down. Enter the tactic of humiliation. And it's actually the humiliation that completely destroyed any sense of self-worth or security in who I was as a boy, and later, attempting to find my way as a man, caused a whole host of issues in my adult life.

I want to make a disclaimer that violence happens across all cultures and walks of life, and while this is my experience, it should not be taken to endorse or perpetuate negative racial stereotyping about a culture and people I hold so dear to my heart. I am proud to be Sāmoan, but I can choose to leave parts of what has become 'culture' due to a range of factors, including colonisation.

Imagine feeling so unsafe that you would not only do the wrong thing, but also be the wrong person. My opinion was unsafe to share. My mistakes were unsafe to make. My fears were unsafe to have. Being *me*, Matt Brown, was unsafe, because at the core of who I was, I was ridiculed and belittled by the people who were first meant to love me.

I wasn't like my older brothers. I was far more introverted. I loved art and music, while my brothers were more into sports. I didn't enjoy having any attention focused on me, so I did my best to stay under the radar. But this was impossible, because I was constantly made to feel different. My body wasn't the same as my brothers' bodies, so I became the laughing stock. Throughout my childhood I was repeatedly stripped naked, mocked and laughed at by my parents.

My extended family would come over to our house, and my Mother would pull my pants down and laugh openly about my genitals. This would instigate ridicule amongst my family, aunties, cousins and uncles. Amidst the very people I was meant to feel safe with, I learnt the meaning of the word 'unsafe'.

I started to feel anxiety (as I now understand it to be) at about four or five years old. At the time I would have described the sensation as a swirling stomach that would make me feel physically sick. As soon as I knew we were having our extended family over, the fear would creep in. I would go and quickly hide either in the wardrobe or under the bed; it was a pointless attempt to delay the inevitable. My parents would make my older brothers go and find me, and they'd drag me into the lounge by my arm or by my legs. This happened repeatedly until I was about nine years old. As I got older, sometimes I'd try to fight my brothers, but they were bigger and stronger than me so it was futile. And if they didn't pull me into the lounge as requested by my Mother, they, too, would have received hidings.

It was their idea of funny. I'd be pulled into the lounge and, while my family all sat around, my brothers would pull my pants down, and take off my clothes. I would stand there naked and crying, trying desperately to cover myself with my hands. It would go for what would seem to be the longest five minutes of my life.

I looked over once to my younger brother, who was staring at me with tears in his eyes. We are the closest in age, with just over a year's difference, and I knew in that moment he felt for me. But there was nothing he could do. I was the son selected for this because my penis was the smallest. That was hilarious apparently; enough so that it gave them years of laughter at my expense.

When, finally, I was told I could go and put my clothes on, I would run out of the room and back to my hiding place, where I'd cry alone.

Humiliation wasn't inflicted only on me. It was just as painful, if not worse, watching my parents publicly shame my brothers. I recall watching one of my older brothers get a particularly nasty hiding from my Father in front of us at home. He was beating my brother with a belt. This was pretty normal, but the next day my brother's eye had bruised up very badly, as the belt buckle had whipped around his face and got caught in his eye. It was one of the worst black eyes I had ever seen. Later that day we had to go over to our Uncle's house (my Father's relative), and us brothers went into our cousin's bedroom immediately.

I eventually made my way into the lounge where my parents were talking to my Uncle. My Father was proudly telling him about how he had given my brother a 'big hiding'. My Uncle was in agreement that this was a good thing, as we needed to be taught a lesson. Then my Uncle said he wanted to see my brother, so he told me to go into my cousin's bedroom to get him. I went in and told him to go into the lounge as Uncle wanted to see him.

He refused and hid under the bed, covering his eye. Hearing of his refusal to comply, my Uncle came into the bedroom and pulled the entire bed away from where my brother was cowering underneath, covering his eye, whimpering. My Uncle then got his belt out and started hitting my brother with it, until he was forced to get up and sit in the lounge where he was ridiculed further.

I was always a sensitive child, and, even though I was only about seven years old at the time, I will never forget what seeing someone else being humiliated like that did to my soul. It was torture to see him be shamed like that and not be able to protect him from it in any way.

Being constantly humiliated as children brought us feelings of extreme unworthiness, helplessness, anxiety and powerlessness. I felt exposed, unprotected, degraded and diminished. Of course, as a young child I didn't have adequate language to explain those feelings, but as an adult I can now pinpoint the feelings because, in all honesty, they have never fully gone away.

'Imagine feeling so unsafe that you would not only do the wrong thing, but also be the wrong person. My opinion was unsafe to share. My mistakes were unsafe to make. My fears were unsafe to have.'

Being humiliated is so utterly confidence-destroying that I can recall what happened in vivid detail now, 20-plus years later. It's like I am right there as the child, stripped naked and being laughed at.

How that humiliation became shame in my life was when what was done to me became who I actually was, and with it came the belief that I was unworthy of love and belonging to anyone. Because of what I had experienced at the hands of significant people to me, I felt – at the deepest place – completely unworthy of connection, and so became emotionally disconnected from all those around me.

I understand how, at this point, the use of alcohol or illegal drugs can become a very real option for many. I have seen this play out with many Brothers, friends and clients. They'll do anything to numb the pain and so self-medicate. Research shows that when we numb our vulnerability, it will manifest in other destructive ways – like addiction, depression, eating disorders, bullying, suicide and violence – because we are also numbing our ability to feel joy, gratitude and happiness.

Like I said, my drug of choice was music. Music of all genres brought me freedom and took me somewhere else. I could put on my headphones and get lost in lyrics and beats that would transport me to another place. Music – and in particular hip-hop – could bring people's stories together and make me feel not quite so alone in the world. Heroes of mine, like Tupac Shakur, shared their stories of pain, survival and abandonment, which made me more able to articulate my experiences. For many of us in the nineties, rappers and musicians became the parents we didn't have. It was like they were raising us while we were barely surviving what was being thrown at us.

I would put headphones on as a teenager and then just walk for hours, alone, across my city. Anything was preferable to being at home. To this day I am grateful to music for saving me in so many ways. As a teenager I was so suicidal and shut down. Many times I seriously considered taking my own life, to the point where I would sometimes sleep on train tracks, wishing desperately that a train would free me from my life while I was sleeping. I felt alone and misunderstood, and I had no one to talk to. It wasn't the pain from the life I had been exposed to that was destroying me either. It was the intense shame that I felt at the deepest level of my existence, and the absolute belief that no one would, or could, ever love me if they actually saw me for who I was. My goal, therefore, became to remain hidden at any cost.

I've learnt from Brené that shame will either tell us that we're never good enough, or ask us **'Who do you think you are?'** Shame tells us that we are mistakes, and we – men in particular – don't want to be seen as weak. By hiding away, I was trying to protect myself, but it didn't work because I shut down so much else inside me. When I first watched Brené speak, I was so impacted by the quotation from former US President Theodore Roosevelt that she shared. The quote goes like this:

> It is not the critic who counts, not the one who points out how the strong man stumbled or how the doer of deeds might have done them better. The credit belongs to the man who is actually in the arena, whose face is marred with sweat and dust and blood; who strives valiantly; who errs and comes short again and again; who knows the great enthusiasms, the great devotions, and spends himself in a worthy cause; who, if he wins, knows the triumph of high achievement; and who, if he fails, at least fails while *daring greatly*, so that his place shall never be with those cold and timid souls who know neither victory nor defeat.

Up to this point, I wasn't someone who had ever given myself the opportunity to 'dare greatly' because of my upbringing, but somewhere along the way I found the courage to leave my stable job as a joiner, where I had been working for nine years, and start up the barbershop in my tin garden shed in Aranui, Christchurch. This was my first arena, and somewhere I found the courage to dare greatly in my own life.

One of the masks I wore constantly was one of lies. My Mother regularly lied, and I could see first-hand that it was all about helping her survive her situation and avoiding abuse. She would always be untruthful with my Father – doing her best to tell him what she thought he wanted to hear, in an attempt to keep his anger at bay. I quickly learnt that if I lied and told others what they wanted to hear, it stopped unwanted connection, and I could do and be whomever I wanted. I thought it helped me appear to be 'cool', even though inside I felt anything but cool. It helped me be someone I wasn't, and it helped me pretend that I wasn't ashamed of who I really was.

And then I met someone who could see through the bullshit. Someone who valued truth and wouldn't accept anything less. Someone who wasn't scared to say things as she saw them.

I met Sarah.

And so some years into our friendship she sat me down one day, looked me in the eye, and said, quietly but firmly, the words that have utterly changed my life: 'Matt, I know that you lie. I can give you clear examples of when you have lied to me if you want, but I want to tell you, as your friend, that you don't need to lie to me anymore. With me you can just be yourself.'

Then she was silent and waited for me to respond.

I was initially speechless, and then, of course, my immediate reaction was to lie.

'What do you mean?' I asked. 'I don't lie to you!'

I remember my heart started pounding, and a flush heated up my face.

'Yes, you do,' she said calmly, and then proceeded to repeat back some of the lies I had told her during our time together as friends. She did so with such calm assurance, I think at that point I knew the show was well and truly over. I couldn't deny it, and she had, indeed, seen through me.

I felt exposed. I wanted to cry. I wanted to run away and hide forever from her and from everyone. I felt like a child. I felt humiliated. I felt ashamed. I felt like she had shamed me. I felt that, because she was triggering these extremely intense feelings of shame, she *was* shame. Suddenly I was the kid being stripped naked in the middle of the lounge being laughed at by her, and I felt angry.

'Listen,' she said. 'I see the real you, and I'm telling you that you don't need to lie to me. I love the real you, and I'm telling you this so you can stop trying to be someone else, and just be yourself with me.'

This took my breath away. She had just said to my face that she saw me – **the real me** – and loved me, and that I didn't need to be anyone else.

The thought was enticing. I thought immediately how it would be much easier to just be honest with her, as lying to be someone else was pretty exhausting and time-consuming, always having to remember what I said. But, on the other hand, I wondered just how much of me she had seen, and surely she wasn't talking about the really bad shameful stuff.

I got that sick feeling in my stomach. If she really knew the worst bits she wouldn't be saying this, I thought. But then, somewhere in my soul, I found a glimmer of hope. If she knew I was a liar and still wanted to be my friend, then maybe – just maybe – I could share some of my most painful feelings with her.

'Oh, the exposure,' I thought, as I was sitting there quietly debating my options internally. To be seen or not to be seen? *That* was the question – but what was the answer?

Ironically, it came back to vulnerability. Because if vulnerability is the most accurate measurement of courage, to let ourselves really be seen, so that we have any kind of shot of love and genuine belonging, then we need to be willing to invest in something where there are no guarantees, and just see what happens. We need to be vulnerable. And trust in it.

So that day I made one of the most defining decisions of my life. Looking at the experiences we had shared so far, I decided she had proved herself to be trustworthy. Sarah had never humiliated me or made jokes at my expense. She was respectful, and had always taken the utmost care with my feelings when I had been insecure. Importantly, unlike the experiences of my childhood, she kept my confidences and didn't later use things I said or did against me. I decided that if I invited her into my heart to walk places no one else had ever been invited into, she was someone who would take her shoes off at the door and tread carefully.

And so I accepted the invitation to show her the real me. As I said earlier, though, it wasn't an overnight thing. I had to be the one doing all the heavy lifting. Sarah's role could only be one of supporting me as I did the actual work of changing and growing. And finding the confidence to do it, and continue on, took time. But it was a start.

It happened in increments. I started telling her things no one else knew. I started telling her about my most shameful moments. And in sharing them, and revisiting those childhood events with the eyes of an adult, I came to realise that sometimes there can be a vast difference between what actually happened to us, and what we believe happened. How we frame events can make so much difference.

Sometimes my feelings of shame meant I couldn't talk, only cry instead. Loud, embarrassing sobs that I had held onto for the longest time.

She would listen to me in such a present, still way, then help me re-frame what to take away from the experience: 'I'm sorry that happened to you, but that was never your fault, and that is not who you are.'

Brick by brick, I took down the walls I had built around myself, and with Sarah's help I learnt that having boundaries was far more effective than building walls. Walls kept everyone out. Establishing boundaries meant that toxic people no longer had the power to humiliate me anymore. When, even as an adult, members of my family made fun of me, or made jokes at my expense, I didn't need to say nothing and put up with it. I didn't need to buy into the old feelings of shame and inadequacy and humiliation they were trying to burden me with.

In reality, I wasn't powerless. I had a choice. It was perfectly okay to tell them 'No', I would not be treated that way, and to teach them how I wanted to be treated. If they still disrespected me, then it was perfectly okay, too, to not continue being in a relationship with them in the same way. They would eventually learn the way I deserved to be treated, and comply, or I wouldn't allow them access to me in the same way I had.

And when I started doing this there was an immediate drop-off in people whose toxicity had always damaged me, but who I'd still allowed into my life. But their going also made room for new kind-hearted souls to come into my life, people who loved me in ways I had always desired to be loved.

In this way, I learnt that you can never really be truly loved until you are seen, and that you are only loved as much as you are known.

ALTHOUGH MY WIFE was never my shame, sometimes her actions or questions would trigger the feelings of shame that I had previously felt. This happens for so many men I know personally. Sometimes my instinctive response to feeling ashamed is to hide

– either by running away or by lying to cover up further. But I've come to understand that when the shame within us is triggered, while it's natural to react or hide, we have to come to the place where we find refuge and still be present. Nor do we hit out at her. She is not our enemy. Our enemy is within ourselves – it is the pain and shame and trauma that is longing to be felt, and seen, and healed.

And the fact that Sarah – my person, my wife, my lover, my soulmate – chooses to sit in the front row, hearing the very worst of what I have to share, means that she has become a source of light for me. Shame cannot possibly exist in the light – it only lives in the dark places we choose to hide it in, in relationships we aren't honest in. By her 'turning the light on', by speaking truth in our friendship, this meant that by the time we came together as a couple and were married, shame had no place at our table, even when it did its best to remind me at times of my unworthiness.

Sarah was never my shame; she was light.

Sarah was also the first person I had consensual intercourse with. After years of sexual abuse from both women and men in my childhood, after being raped by my Uncle, after experiencing endless humiliation, being ridiculed and laughed at naked – well, being sexually intimate with someone as a grown adult wasn't something I felt I wanted at all. In fact, I was terrified.

For about a year when I was 19, I'd had a relationship of sorts with a close male friend. We'd met while living in a boys' home together, where most of us had come from similar backgrounds. Because this guy and I also worked together, we were often in close proximity to each other, and sexual touching of sorts became an extension of our close friendship and bond. Because of the sexual violation I had experienced in my childhood I felt confused and conflicted about my own sexuality, while also yearning for male connection because of the lack of a relationship with my Father. At this point in my life, this friendship felt safe, and it became safe to explore in a consensual way the inevitable sexual desires of a teenage boy. There was an innocence that we shared, in a way.

Now, when I look back at this season, I observe that teenage Matt automatically sexualised a safe connection, because he had never had one, and so didn't know how else to express love and gratitude to my friend. Now, more than 15 years later, I understand that we can be close to people and connect with them on a deep level without feeling the need to sexualise the relationship.

Our relationship ran its course, and we mutually felt that this wasn't what we wanted for our lives. So we ended the sexual component, but thankfully stayed close friends, after negotiating the initial awkward period following the change in our relationship.

'Being humiliated is so utterly confidence-destroying that I can recall what happened in vivid detail now, 20-plus years later. It's like I am right there as the child, stripped naked and being laughed at.'

From then on I truly believed, with the religious beliefs of my upbringing, that it would be better to be as celibate as a monk, and perhaps even locked up in a monastery, far away from anyone who could hurt me. The thought of ever being exposed again, and opening myself up to another – with the potential for that relationship ending – was too much for me, and so for a long time in my early twenties I shut myself away from everyone and became very guarded. When I met my future wife at age 24, I told her in genuine sincerity that 'God has called me to celibacy'. The truth was I was frightened of my own sexuality, and fearful of what any kind of true intimacy would potentially do.

Eventually with my wife I learnt the huge difference between being exposed and being transparent. One was forced access by them, and the other was granted access by me. I had given her a swipe-card to my soul with an 'all-access pass'. When it was time to get physically naked, she had already seen my soul. The feelings of safety that came from being truly seen, accepted and loved meant that when I was naked I was unashamed. The overwhelming feeling afterwards was a mixture of liberation and a vulnerability hangover. I ended up going into the bathroom, and crying tears for a little boy who finally felt safe to be seen.

All those years before, when I was stripped naked and laughed at, I had told myself afterwards, in my moments crying under the bed, that the essence of who I was was ugly, unlovable, laughable, unworthy. I felt I wasn't deserving of belonging. My shame and humiliation separated me from those who tried to get close to me in subsequent years. But nothing I did to hide my shame over the years succeeded in eradicating it. That is, until I did the opposite. I faced it.

The thing I thought I could never do, I did with her.

That day in our bedroom I dared greatly. Shame lost and love won.

Love told me something different, something new. It said: 'You were so worried about being seen? Darling boy, you have to be seen to be loved, and here you are, naked and loved.'

Chapter five

She is not your trauma

FOR CENTURIES, IT HAS BEEN SAID 'to the defiled all things are defiled'. This means that the trauma, or the 'defilement' inside ourselves, is how we then see everything else in our world. In that regard, the world - and the people in our world - are an external mirror into our inner reality.

World-renowned author and expert on the connection between childhood trauma and addiction, and a hero of mine, Dr Gabor Maté, says: 'Trauma is not what happens to you. Trauma is what happens inside of you as a result of what happens to you.'

The traumatised, the defiled and the unhealed often seem to be drawn to the same kind of abuse or dysfunction that once traumatised them. But why on earth would we be attracted to something we hate so much and wouldn't wish on anyone else? It is because, I believe, we have bonded with the trauma, and it has become such a normal part of our existence that we often mistake this abuse or dysfunction for love.

Psychologist Dr Nicole LePera writes: 'The most overlooked addiction is the addiction to another human being where you can act out the dysfunction of your childhood.' These are the 'trauma bonds' or 'betrayal bonds' that represent 'the misuse of fear, excitement, sexual feelings, and sexual physiology'. This terminology was first introduced by Dr Patrick Carnes in 1997, and applies to relationships where there is an exploitation of trust or power.

This is also when we repeat the same dynamics we first experienced in childhood with our parents or caregivers, but later carry them on ourselves with our romantic partners, or sometimes with really close friends. The harmful underlying theme is that **we must betray ourselves in order to receive love**.

We may have had a relationship with our parents that was unpredictable, where a huge imbalance of power existed, and which moved quickly between moments of cruelty, abuse and dysfunction, and moments of love and tenderness. It's confusing because the people who say they love us, or seem loving at times, were often really hurting us.

So it's no accident that, when we finally escape our own toxic childhoods – if we haven't healed enough to turn our wounds into scars – we simply attract more of the same kind of dysfunction, abuse and violence that we say (and truly believe) that we don't want.

Having come from a life exactly like this, and talking to countless men all day from similar backgrounds for over a decade now, I can wholeheartedly say most of us have not got a single clue about this stuff. We have no awareness of why we've gone from bad relationship to bad relationship. One Brother I was talking with the other day said to me: 'I've always just ended up with the same as what I had, but I don't even want that! I just don't know how to get better.'

More than anything, with all the work, writing, education and advocacy I now do – especially with men – my deepest desire is to show that a very different life *is* possible to the traumatised souls who, like me, were once abused and degraded so horrifically that it was hard to even imagine a life beyond living in a traumatised state.

I do not believe that violent abusers are born that way, because the reality I've seen myself is that they are made - moulded by years of trauma, neglect and a lack of access to adequate mental healthcare and empathy. A huge majority of the violent men I have had the honour to speak with are, in fact, victims themselves - often as a result of prolonged and intergenerational abuse. This is trauma that repeats itself for generations, until someone has the courage to stand up and say: 'This shit ends with me!' If you have the courage to do the work in healing what is intensely painful, you have the power of healing your family line.

Hiding our problems has never ever healed them. In fact, the complete opposite is true: they fester in the dark, so our wounds become infected, and spread infection throughout our bodies and on to more bodies. I have discovered that angry, violent men are often traumatised little boys living in adults' bodies, because, like I repeatedly say: **what we refuse to transform, we will inevitably transmit.**

'Trauma bonds imitate the first relationships we saw or had when we were children. It's where we repeat cycles of behaviour that are familiar to us – even if that behaviour hurts us and hurts our partner.'

So, keeping in mind what trauma is, and the inevitable damage to our mind, body and spirit that occurs from a single traumatic event (like being raped one night), or a series of repeated traumatic events (like living with domestic violence for your entire childhood), this damage then manifests itself - usually via our emotions, and how we react to those we live with.

So now you can fully imagine two of these traumatised individuals, bonded together, attempting to somehow have a healthy, functional relationship – only to discover it's just not working. It saddens me greatly how normal it is to see relationships that are simply based on trauma bonds. Trauma bonds imitate the first relationships we saw or had when we were children. It's where we repeat cycles of behaviour that are familiar to us – even if that behaviour hurts us and hurts our partner.

Late one night, I was having a heart-to-heart conversation with Sarah, as we were making sense of the definitions of co-dependency and gaining clarity on trauma bonds. She was sharing about a past relationship she'd had when she was only a teenager, with a man more than a decade older than her. I knew all about it. It hadn't been a respectful relationship at all, and he had been an addict of multiple substances. That night I asked her what lessons she took away from that relationship, and how they had helped her awareness and growth in our relationship now.

She was initially quiet and very reflective. Then she started talking about an earlier childhood experience that immediately came to mind.

I'll let her share this, so that you can understand from a woman's perspective how this kind of relationship bonded on trauma plays out.

> A distinctive memory from my childhood is how my parents would discipline me. If my adoptive Mother deemed me to be disobedient, or if I misbehaved during the day, she would tell me to wait until my adoptive Father got home. This meant I would spend the entire rest of the day anxious, with a sick feeling of dread in my stomach, awaiting the inevitable punishment to come. It was always the same. When he arrived home he was never in the best mood after work anyway, because he worked long hours for a minimum wage in a job he didn't particularly enjoy. There was very little joy about his life, and, looking back, I think he lived his life in permanent frustration – so after work was never really a good time.

> My heart would be pounding fast. I would often need to go to the toilet from my upset tummy. I would hear her tell him in hushed tones what I had done, and he would come down to my bedroom and shut the door behind him. He would sit on the edge of my bed and face me while I stood in front of him.
>
> He would stare at me, repeat back what he had been told, and tell me to pull my pants down till I was half naked. I would then have to bend over and he would spank my ass, either with his hand, a wooden spoon or his belt. He would stop once I would admit defeat and cry. I hated that. I never wanted to cry. I just wanted it to be over. He would then pull me up and sit me on his lap and tell me he did this because he loved me. He loved me so much he had to discipline me, he said.

It always hurts me to think of anyone hurting her as a child. 'What do you think that set you up to believe?' I asked.

> I guess, to get to the part where he loved me, I had to be hurt first. Love was always interwoven with hurt and shame. The shame of pulling my pants down and standing there in front of him like that, and the shame of having to cry, so he knew he was effective in hurting me. I hated those parts the most, but you had to go through them to get to the bit where he loved you, and then it was almost a relief.
>
> Usually if I had been punished like this, my adoptive Father would be in a good mood afterwards – more than he usually would be after work – because he was often very short-tempered and impatient with us. So, in this way, I grew up thinking it was better for everyone. He could take out his frustrations on me, and we'd all have a nicer Father for the rest of the night.

'So you believed that him doing this to you was the best for everyone?' I asked. 'When did you come up with that assumption?'

Not initially, I don't think. I was really young when punishments like this started. I was punished like this for as long as I can remember, but I know I was always quite aware of everything, and very perceptive of my environment and the dynamics of the relationships around me.

As I got older, I knew for sure that I hated that uneasy sick feeling of dread in my stomach that came before being punished, so any prolonged periods of uncertainty in my own life I hate even now. That feeling is the worst!

I had various relationships all through my teenage years. They weren't particularly bad – I was just young and so naïve! I never really let anyone in on an emotionally intimate level, so they only went so far. I was so scared of being rejected that I wouldn't allow myself to be in any sort of position to ever be rejected. We had fun, and that was it. So all my relationships were casual, not super-committed, or really involved on a deep level.

I met him when I was 19 years old, and he was 30. I was attracted to him immediately – but I was also attracted to his wider family dynamic. I yearned for a loving family so desperately, and since I left home at 15 I guess I had spent time looking for this. I met him at a family dinner my friend had taken me to. She was friends with his brother. I think a lot of my usual walls came down quickly. I thought his family seemed so lovely, so he must be, too. When he contacted me to hang out it went from 0 to 100 so quickly – I didn't realise that he was just coming out of a long-term relationship where he had a three-year-old son. I had no idea how this was going to play out for me.

I fell pregnant to him almost straight away, and emotionally bonded to someone who still loved someone else. In the early days of being pregnant, I rocked around to his Mother's house one morning before work, and I walked in on him and his ex-girlfriend asleep naked in bed together from a night out.

It was like someone had thrown a huge bucket of ice-cold water over my head. I snuck out, didn't confront them, and went to work in shock. I didn't know what to do. I knew I didn't want this. But it hurt that he didn't want me. Or he wanted someone else more than me. This didn't help with the extreme feelings of rejection and unworthiness I had already always felt.

This is when the cycle started for me. The trauma bond. I would do whatever was required to be chosen by him.

There was so much hurt and shame. And then he would say he was sorry and that he loved me. There I was, back on my Father's lap having him tell me he loved me after he had just beaten me half-naked.

It went round and round like that for the whole nine months of my pregnancy. One day he loved me, and he was charming and nice to me. I even moved into his Mother's house with him. I loved his family so much, so that was half of his appeal. The next day he was yelling abuse at me, trying to smash my car windows with a baseball bat, coming down off a high, telling me I was the fattest girl he had ever been with.

He was always out partying, constantly unfaithful, and spent all the savings I had worked so hard for. He had so much hurt and unresolved trauma of his own. He would transmit all of it onto me.

I would cry and cry, pregnant, young and alone, utterly clueless as to how this all worked. If it was really bad, I would go stay at a friend's house for a few nights, but inevitably he would call, and sweet-talk his way back in. I would always just want to get to that good bit, so I'd move through all the hurt and shame just to get to that place where the physical chemistry was always amazing, and he would tell me he loved me and promise he would do better. If I could just help him and love him, he would change, he promised.

In the times when it was good, I would tell myself I just had to do whatever it took to love him well. I could love him back to life. I truly believed that. I could love him through his insecurities, his addictions and hurt from his previous relationship. He needed to be physically desired by as many women as possible to feel validated. Deep down I knew that I was never really enough for what he needed.

But I would sit there listening to 'our' song, 'By Your Side' by Sade. I would picture our wedding, as I would sing those words to myself on repeat – words about never leaving your lover's side, no matter what.

No, I wouldn't leave his side – even if he had no intention of ever committing to me. I'd do anything except leave him, including sacrificing myself. I knew how it felt to have people who would love you and leave you, so I would not do that to anyone, ever. This roller-coaster of emotions that were ever-changing, day to day, happened right up until I gave birth.

It was the birth of our precious daughter that woke me up.

It was my first taste of love. Real love. The constant, consistent love of a first-time Mother for her child – someone part of me already. The night after I came home from the hospital with our baby, he didn't come home. I knew where he was. He didn't have to tell me. He had stayed with his ex-girlfriend again, and it was in this exact moment I knew, without doubt, I didn't want our daughter to see this chaos masquerading as a relationship.

I never doubted he loved our daughter. But I knew what I was experiencing with him was not the love I really desired. So I packed up my little two-door car with my baby and all her things, and left the very next day to move in with a friend.

I wish I could say that it ended there. It didn't. I didn't live with him, but he still had access to me for the next year or so. He would come and visit me at night after the baby was asleep. Sometimes he would stay with me. When he did, he was so physically affectionate that I pretended he loved me, because he was there with me, wasn't he?

On other nights he stayed with his ex and his son. The remaining nights he would be partying with friends and staying God only knows where, so the situation essentially worked exactly how he wanted. He had the freedom to go wherever, and to whomever, he wanted.

The situation wasn't working well for me at all. Having no family support of my own, with a new baby and all that entailed, bonded with a guy who was uncommitted to our day-to-day life, but who popped by when he wanted, meant that the extreme feelings of rejection and unworthiness would completely take me over. I got to the point where I attempted to take my life by overdosing on sedatives when my daughter was only seven months old.

It was all just too much. I was literally hanging on for dear life to just be loved, and all that we had were these crazy waves of emotional abuse, times of heated conflict and drama, and then the inevitable non-committed sex. It was so far from the love I know now.

It wasn't until our daughter was 18 months old that it all stopped. By then I had my first house – just for the two of us. We had a Christmas party. I invited him. I knew he would expect to stay, but I was tired of that and, by now, I was stronger. I had already decided I wouldn't let him stay, and when the time came I told him to go home with his sister. He was almost shocked. He didn't like it. But I was firm. I had decided.

'This isn't how this is going to be anymore. I don't want that for her or for me. Let's just leave it at that.'

It wasn't even a discussion. I knew I was done with self-sabotaging my own life. I had started to heal, too. Having the courage to live alone does that to you.

He was reluctant to leave, but he did, and I was never intimate with him ever again after that. He tried a few times, but I was so focused on my own journey and healing by then that I truly wasn't even interested. I felt sad for our daughter that I couldn't give her the perfect family, with two parents together, but I vowed I would give her a healed Mother.

It took years and years of healing. I would cry by myself in the car so she wouldn't hear me and get upset. I worked through all my pain and grief, sadness and fears of always being unloved and rejected. I grieved the loss of what I really wanted, but wasn't going to get from those I wanted to give it to me. I told myself that I could give to myself what no one had ever given to me. I practised daily how to love myself, and show up for myself, and how to keep my word to myself, and make the dreams inside my heart happen. It was endless tears and years dedicated to self-work.

When I walked up the aisle to you, Matt, at 5 p.m. on 29 August 2015, I knew, without doubt, that this was everything I had healed for. My daughter, now 12 years old, sang me up the aisle to 'our song' – the one that described everything about our journey into wholeness, and into love.

It was 'Beneath Your Beautiful' by Emeli Sandé and Labrinth. In stark contrast to 'By Your Side', the lyrics were about loving a strong woman, a woman who has been through so much, for exactly who she is.

The walls of trauma inside of us had come crashing down and here we were. My daughter became our daughter, and she witnessed first-hand the miracle of what the bonds of trauma looked like when shattered.

They had lost their power.

Remember – Dr Gabor Maté says: **'Trauma is not what happens to you. Trauma is what happens inside of you as a result of what happens to you.'**

I want to add that healing is not what happens *to* you. Healing is what happens *inside* of you as a result of what love does to you.

Yes, trauma can scar you and make you less flexible, more rigid, and feel like you always have to live on the defence. It never, ever serves us well because it closes down our willingness and ability to feel.

When we decide to, we can each choose a new path. One that requires us to open up and be vulnerable. It's not easy, but when you have the courage to work through the old story that for too long has held you bound, then healing happens. One day when you can move through the pain, through all the old patterns, and decide that you will change the narrative to create a new story, this is when our childhood trauma no longer keeps us bound.

Is it time now, Brother, to begin your own journey of healing?

Chapter six

She is not your saviour

SAVIOUR: A PERSON WHO SAVES someone else.

My Brothers, I'm going to keep it real here and be very specific: no matter how hard she tries, she *cannot* save you from yourself.

She cannot save you from your demons, your addictions, your drama, your pain, your shame or your bad habits - none of it! It is just not her shit to save you from, and it never will be her responsibility.

And for all my Sisters who are sneakily reading this book hoping to glean some insight, please do not spend another second of your life attempting to redirect a man from a path he has chosen to walk down. He has nothing to lose in you doing this, and you have absolutely everything about yourself to lose in the process of trying to save him. Think of it as if he's in the ocean drowning and you jump in *unable to swim* but trying valiantly to save him! You are so far out of your depth. And neither of you will make it to the safety of the shore.

Women can inspire us to want to be better, yes, but save us and make us better? Hell no!

She cannot save you, she cannot fix you, and she cannot rescue you from what is, inevitably, the outcome of the choices and decisions you have made, or not made, for your life.

She might *really* want to. I've met countless women who want to save their men so badly. And if saving us actually depended on *how much* they want to save us, then - trust me - we'd all be saved.

Many women have made it their life's mission to invest in our 'potential' - the qualities or abilities we all have within us that *may* be developed, and which *could* lead to possible success. We are all born with potential. Some of us do the work in realising that potential, to actually manifest it in real life. Others do nothing with that potential, and hope that someone like her will swoop in and do the work for them to make their potential a reality.

Put simply, what does 'doing the work' look like?

It looks like accepting the following:

1. She is not responsible for *your* emotional rehabilitation.

2. Your healing is *your* responsibility, and yours to take the initiative on and manage.

3. Any healing needed for you cannot come at the expense of her healing, health and wellbeing.

4. She can support you, but she can never do more for you than you are prepared to do for yourself.

5. Regardless of what anyone has done *to you*, it is now time *for you* to take ownership of your own life, and be committed to living it wholeheartedly enough to do any work needed. Your childhood trauma wasn't your fault, but your healing is now your responsibility.

6. True change comes from genuine growth. Growth happens once we heal. Healing starts when we begin to *feel* our pain.

7. Hurt people invariably hurt people, because what we do not transform, we transmit on to those around us. Healed people do indeed heal people.

The question is: will you have the courage to heal?

The men who sit back and wait to be saved by a good woman are also the victims who blame people like her when it doesn't work out. You know the type: it's always someone else's fault why it's not working out for him.

Do you get how crazy that is? How can she really do the work for you when you won't? I know that most women are well intentioned, too; they want the best for our lives, and the lives of our children, so they think they'll just 'help us out' in this little area, because...

If only he could just get past this...
If only he could just change this little thing...
If only he could see himself how I see him...
No one has ever loved him how I love him...
He's had such a hard life...
If I don't do this, who will?

You will!

Or you won't.

But either way, Brothers, it is absolutely our time to say, with resolve, that *we* will.

We will be responsible for saving ourselves.

We will be responsible for finding new tools and learning new ways to help ourselves heal.

We will be responsible for our own lives.

And if we refuse to take responsibility, then we must live with the consequences that our lack of action delivers.

I've met so many men who simply don't want to do the work. They want a better life than the one they have currently, yet they refuse to do the work it takes to improve their life.

It makes no sense to expect better but do nothing.

And far too often women come along and rescue men from their own responsibility because they so badly want them to have this better life. She rationalises it as: 'It'll be better for me if he's better himself.'

I want to share with you a story about a woman I know. Every man she's ever been in a relationship with has thought she could save them. Her belief in the man, and her willingness to support him to become a better person, is invariably mistaken by the man to be an offer that she will take over and do all the work for him! And when this well-meaning woman realises she has been given the rough end of the bargain, she tries to stick it out in the belief that 'he will change'.

But I want to humanise the woman behind the alias of Saviour, so that you *really* understand the physical and emotional cost to a woman of trying to save a man who, in reality, doesn't want saving enough to do anything about it himself.

My friend grew up as the daughter of a man who wasn't affectionate at all. He struggled with his own mental health, and was so emotionally distant and uninvolved with her life that she would say now she barely knows him as an adult, even though her parents are still together, and she lived with them both until she left home at 16 years of age.

He didn't interact with her much, and when he did it was with humorous little put-downs and jokes at her expense that left her thinking very little of herself. She is now in her thirties, a single Mother with four children. By the time she left home, she was yearning for love and craving affection. The problem was, because of what she lacked in a relationship with her Father, her self-worth was lacking considerably, too. So she threw herself into relationships with men who were never her equals, because she really didn't hope for too much. What she did hope was that her efforts to 'help him to be better' would mean that he would then be in a better position to love her in the way she wanted.

I spoke with her recently, at the conclusion of her third serious relationship, and asked her what she had learned. She said she realised she had spent half her life investing so much in 'his' potential that she didn't have much energy left for her own.

I asked her why she had spent so much of herself and her life investing in men, when they hadn't invested in themselves.

They certainly hadn't invested anything in her or her potential – in fact, they had actually hindered her growth massively.

She was quiet for a long while before she answered me. Finally she said that she knew what it was like to not be given a chance, so she wanted to give him the chance she felt no one had ever given her. She also admitted that she had stayed in the relationship when she had wanted to leave five years before. For five years she had stayed, and for five years she had invested in something that never really paid off for either of them. He was an addict then, and is still an addict today. His financial instability, substance abuse, depression, abusive behaviour directed at her, and his own childhood issues that left him wounded, were all dumped in her lap to have to live with and sort through.

'She cannot save you, she cannot fix you, and she cannot rescue you from what is, inevitably, the outcome of the choices and decisions you have made, or not made, for your life.'

Not only did the investment of her time, emotional energy, and even her finances not pay off, but it cost her even more in reduced confidence, poor mental health, and her own lost years. She had just delayed the inevitable by not leaving when she first knew she should.

When he was with her she would cover up certain aspects of his behaviour from others, or collude with his excuses for his behaviour. He never sought adequate help because he didn't need to. He had her managing all the consequences, so he didn't really have to feel a thing.

Often saviours like her go from one man in need of saving to the next – riding into each new relationship to save the day. In the initial stages of the relationship, of course it feels nice to have someone care for you so much, and want to help you by doing so much for you, especially things that you have struggled with for a while now, and even more so if you weren't nurtured by someone properly as a child.

But as time goes by, the inevitable happens, and she will start feeling resentful for doing so much, and not getting the return she is expecting from you. You also start to feel somewhat powerless, because, at your core, you know you aren't taking responsibility for yourself so there's no real growth or progress being made.

I've also learnt that, sometimes, beyond her conscious awareness, her rescuing behaviour is really her trying to repair the damaged sense of herself that developed in childhood. By saving others she is hoping to somehow save herself, but her choice of a man – and how that man eventually treats her – is often history repeating itself, and she ends up with even more damage, reopening wounds that were inflicted on her in childhood. It's not just a cliché when you hear that women often date their Fathers.

Ultimately, rather than saving him as she hoped, this repetition leaves her feeling defeated and even more like a failure, and in a vulnerable state with someone who is so consumed in his own shit that he can't even see hers. Then, when he doesn't understand what he has to start with, a man with no sense of ownership or personal responsibility soon loses interest in her and often moves on when another saviour swoops in.

Brothers, these saviours are very real people. They have been our Mothers, and now our partners, and if we don't make conscious changes they will be our own daughters, attempting to heal themselves from the brokenness that our brokenness inflicts on them.

These women carry the burdens and pay the cost *themselves*, and consequently it affects their ability to be a Mother. If she is diminished, how do you think this plays out when she attempts to give anything to our children? We have to stop pretending she is disposable, or that her time and energy aren't valuable. We have to start humanising her into a being who cannot thrive while she is so undervalued and overworked. We are not her responsibility or a project to fix. Do not allow her to do things for you that you need to do for yourself. Remember, all you will do is delay the inevitable process of having to do this yourself.

I received this letter online recently through one of my social media channels. It stilled my heart, and as I wrote her a response I wondered what I would say if I had the opportunity to write a letter to her partner. Here's what she wrote:

> Matt, I write to you empty.
>
> 24 years old with 2 kids who's gone back and forward to the same abusive guy since I was 16 years old. I'm tired and I feel lifeless.
>
> If you could please give me some words to tell myself when I'm tempted to go back to him (like I have the million damn times before) I promise you I'll read them every day. I've read everything I can find you've written, and your words make me feel stronger.
>
> There's good things about him – there always are, right? He's never hit our children or physically hurt them in any way. And there are reasons he is the way he is that make me so badly want to save him from himself. But there's nothing fucking good when you can't even see out of your eyes because you can't open them, because the hiding is so bad you can't even drive the kids to school.
>
> That's been our life for too long.
>
> I left him (again) in the middle of last week. One night he got so angry he threw his plate of dinner at my head so hard I fell over. Then he was on me, choking me. At dinnertime in front of our kids. This was because he said dinner was shit and I said: 'If you don't like it, don't eat it.'
>
> I passed out when he was choking me and woke up to the kids standing above me in their pyjamas crying and yelling my

> name. He had taken off and left me like that with them.
>
> My almost-8-year-old later said to me: 'Mama, why does Dad hate you so much? I think he wants to kill you.' She wasn't crying now but shaking uncontrollably.
>
> This breaks me the fuck down!
>
> When he apologises, I want to believe every word he says so badly. Because over the years I've told myself I stay for them – her and her little brother. I never had a Dad so I want to give them that at least. Now I don't know what I have to give them at all.

I did reply to her, but I could tell that her partner was the one who really needed to hear from me. Here's what I decided I wanted *him* to know:

> Dear Brother,
>
> I'm saddened to hear that you left the Mother of your children for dead like that in front of your children. Those who feel dead inside can often do unspeakable acts, but to leave your young children alone with their Mother, not knowing if she was alive or dead, tells me of a great emptiness or void inside of you, Brother.
>
> My encouragement to you today is to sit with this emptiness, and ask yourself if this feeling inside of you is something you want to gift to your children.
>
> If it's not, then ask yourself if your treatment of their Mother is gifting them emptiness or love.
>
> I'm grateful you have never physically violated them. This tells me, at some level, you want to do your best to protect them from pain, and it tells me something about the way you view

them – precious people to be taken care of. So I wonder if you would consider thinking about how they see their Mother. About how important she is to them – someone precious, too.

I once heard a quote that resonated with me. The Dalai Lama said: 'Our prime purpose in this life is to help others. And if you can't help them, at least don't hurt them.'

Why this resonates with me, Brother, is because many of us who have been hurt or defiled in our own abuse, then go on to hurt and abuse others. I don't believe we start out to do this intentionally, but because the pain inside us is so great, if it is not transformed or healed, it will be transmitted by default on to those closest to us. Pain demands to be felt. It demands to be expressed. So sometimes, Brother, we need to pause for a bit, and learn to express our pain in ways that are safe for those around us, and safe for us, too.

Pause and breathe. Take some time out to heal the inside of yourself before you hurt those you actually care about. If you can't help the Mother of your children, then at least don't hurt her the same way you have been. Because sadly, your pain is now hurting your children – the most precious people to you.

Today I speak life into the lifeless parts of you, Brother.

The parts of you that no one's seen in a long time.

The parts you haven't seen in a long time.

The parts you aren't sure are even still there.

The parts in you that want to give up.

The parts that choke life out of other people.

The parts that sometimes believe it would be easier to end things.

The parts of you that think running away will fix everything.

There is nowhere to run, and nowhere to hide, Brother. Everywhere you go, you take the pain with you.

Our pain can be our way through.

My life shows this is true. Once I was like one of your children, afraid and shaken. All I ever wanted was for Mum to be safe from Dad. If she was safe, so were we. Our story went on too long because my Mum didn't know she could leave. She tried so hard for years to save my Dad from his pain. All that happened was his pain became her pain, and that became our pain.

As kids, we didn't know what to do with their pain. Some of us tried to numb it with substances, some took this pain and transmitted it onto their partners, and I took the pain and repeatedly attempted to harm myself and take my life.

I wish Dad had the understanding of all this, and the courage to save us from his pain by healing it. Sadly, he still hasn't really – he's just become too old to transmit his pain, so he drinks it away.

But it's not too late for you, Brother. I invite you to understand that the best apology for your children is your changed behaviour that they and their Mother must witness over an extended period of time from you. This will tell them it's safe to be around you. It will require consistent effort from you, my Brother, and will require you reaching out to people who can help transform your pain instead of transmit it. I wish you courage in this. It won't be easy, but it really will be worth the sacrifice.

She can't save you, Brother. You are the only one who can do this.

What an opportunity you have, Brother.

Your pain can stop with you!

You can heal your family line when you heal yourself.

Heal, my Brother, so your children don't have to.

Matt

Ask yourself this:

- How do I start taking responsibility for saving myself?

- How do I find new tools and new ways to help myself heal?

- How do I become responsible for my life?

- How do I deal with the consequences of not taking any action?

WHEN I THINK OF SARAH, and the role she has played in my own healing journey, I am beyond thankful that she had the insight from her own self-work not to rescue me from myself. I'm thankful she *supported* my growth as a man, from an abused boy who could have very easily manipulated her. She *supported* my journey, she's attended counselling sessions with me at times, and she recommended books and courses that she had already found success in, but *she didn't ever once take away my own empowerment.* She trusted me, and the process, and knew that I would find the right answers in my own time, and in my own way.

Sometimes our conversations or realisations have not been easy, but they have always been truthful, and based in reality. She's had the courage to end or redefine relationships where she wasn't celebrated but was merely tolerated – this was a big encouragement to me in my own quest for better balance in relationships of abuse or dysfunction from family members.

I've had clients tell me: 'It's easy for you, Bro, your wife is a good one who actually helps you and understands your process. Mine is *[insert problem here]*, and if she was like Sarah, then things would be different for me!'

To be honest with you, I think that's bullshit. It's just an excuse. I believe we attract what we allow, and we attract a partner to where we are in our lives because our significant other becomes a mirror for the things we need to work on within ourselves. The best help Sarah has been in my path of healing is actually *not* trying to save me, but instead allowing me to clearly see myself.

I've seen women in my own family over the years being expected to step in and 'rescue' their man, being expected to repeatedly do things for their partners that he really needed to do for himself. I've sat with staff whose partners are there to support them, but end up talking for him because he's switched off. Rescuing him is only ever a quick and temporary fix that just ends up being a far longer, harder process for them both!

Individual healing is a process you can't be saved from either.

If she is saving you, it immediately puts your relationship of equality at a disadvantage. She is not your saviour because she is your friend. Friendship is a relationship that goes both ways, and having that at the core of our marriage is what I believe has made our partnership as strong as it is. Our relationship is one where we continually learn to show up for each other in new ways. Sarah says she is not encouraged or inspired by my potential, but by how I realise and actualise my own potential to be the reality of our life together.

Every single one of us has potential.

The question is:

Will we have the courage to heal ourselves, and be able to live as the people we were born to be?

Chapter seven

She is not your ex

GONE ARE THE DAYS where the majority of us marry the first woman we date. Now we are settling down into family life much older than we once did, and having had far more relationships before we eventually commit to 'the one'.

So by the time we are with 'the one' we are likely to have already dated a range of people, lived in other relationships and slept with other women who it didn't work out with. The list of reasons why it didn't work out is potentially endless; however, in all of this, we are indisputably learning about love and conflict.

What I wonder is: *are we learning well?*

Because of the culture of endless choice and availability, many men I know are seeing women back-to-back, and often – because they haven't given themselves time to adequately heal from past relationships – they project a whole range of emotions about an ex-partner onto a current partner. I see men packing up their baggage and just moving it around from woman to woman.

It all seems fun until we arrive before the woman we really want to be with and commit to, and we unload on her a whole host of things we've carried from past relationships. We naïvely think that, because she loves us so much, she also has the skillset to navigate through some heavy shit that isn't hers to unpack.

If you haven't adequately done the work in ending a past relationship properly, and haven't given yourself enough time and space to heal after a break-up, then - *boom!* - your current partner can now become your ex, and, if your relationship lasts at all, with you projecting other people onto her (and chances are it won't), then it will be filled with unnecessary conflict.

Let's think about a few examples, which are all very real to men I know well:

YOUR VERY FIRST LOVE
Possibly a high-school sweetheart, or the girl who got away. This is the girl we had a relationship with when we were much younger and probably a little too naïve to know what love was. In your mind she will probably always be 'the perfect girl', because, I believe, a first love forever imprints on your life and heart in ways that no one else does. Her role is also hugely romanticised, and trust me when I say the dream of her is probably far better than the actual reality of her.

No current partner can ever compete with a romanticised dream of what could have been, versus what actually is. I believe that the people we have any form of relationship with come into your life for a reason, a season, or a lifetime - and most are not here for a lifetime. Be grateful for whatever role she played in your life, and the lessons you received from her, but feel comfortable with leaving her where she belongs - firmly in your past. For whatever reason, you aren't still together - she is not with you now, and now is where you live.

THE ONE WHO BETRAYED YOU
Maybe she was unfaithful, or maybe she somehow breached your confidence. However she betrayed your trust, it can have affected you in many ways, and be affecting your current relationship

if you haven't adequately healed from the hurt that someone betraying you brings.

I've been asked so many times: 'How can I really trust anyone again?' The truth is that trust is built over time, and trust really comes down to our ability to be vulnerable with another. That in itself seems so risky! Especially if we are still feeling bruised from a previous betrayal.

What I have learnt to do, as someone whose trust has been previously violated, is to school myself up on what trust really is, and then how to navigate around giving it to people - especially in close relationships. Not everyone is worthy of our trust, and that is honestly why it is so much better to start any new relationship slowly. No one - I repeat, *no one* - deserves all our trust in every area immediately. Trust is best given in small increments. When someone is faithful with a small amount of what you trust them with, then you can start to trust them with more.

You have the right to be with someone now who actually understands they have to earn your trust before you completely give them your heart, or want to share your life. In saying that, though, you have to check yourself: is it really your current partner or her actions that are untrustworthy now, or are you just being lied to by echoes from your past, and your feelings, which are not always accurate?

If hurt from a past betrayal causes you to believe now that you really can trust no one, then there is definitely healing to be done for you in this area. The reality is you will need to learn how to allow yourself to be vulnerable, to be powerless. This is not an emotion we men want to feel, but remind yourself that you did, in fact, survive the past betrayal, and that - ultimately - it was an opportunity of growth for you.

THE ONE WHO BROKE UP WITH YOU
No one likes rejection, and most men enjoy a chase - especially when their pride has been challenged. The problem with us men is that when our ego takes a knock we can over-compensate in an area to mask the lack of confidence we feel. I've known men who

after being dumped take it so personally that they question their manhood, and have to sleep with multiple women to validate themselves.

I've also known men who just won't take 'No' for an answer, and then take it to a whole new level, becoming a crazy obsessive stalker who won't get it in his head that she doesn't want to be with him. I mean, how dare she not be with this crazy guy who reacts so badly when told 'No'?

The saddest example, though, is when I see a man who refuses to commit properly to a good woman, all because he doesn't want to be in the position of being rejected or dumped ever again. So he sleeps with her when he wants to, and basically does everything that couples do in a relationship, but he won't actually call their relationship what it is. Like not labelling it somehow means he's safer. To me, you've rejected the relationship before she can reject you – but because you have never actually given it a proper chance, you will never know the heights of where it could go. This could be *the* great love story of your life, but you have never given it the energy it needs to grow!

Here's a truth I have learnt about rejection. Not everyone will like you, love you, get you, or want to be with you. You just aren't right for everyone – and it's better you know you aren't right for someone early on.

Imagine yourself standing in front of a vending machine. Inside it is filled with every variety of chocolate bar imaginable. You only have $2, so you can only pick one. Of course, you pick the one you want and like the most. I'm a Snickers bar guy, but my brother is a Crunchie bar guy. A Snickers isn't necessarily better than a Crunchie, it's just what I personally like best. I'm not deliberately rejecting the others in the vending machine – I just want the Snickers, so it's the obvious choice for me to spend the two bucks I have on the one that I want the most.

Sometimes in life you are the one who, for whatever reason, doesn't get picked, or are told that you aren't wanted. It does hurt – especially when it's in a relationship that you have been invested in. But please remember this vending machine. Not everyone standing in front of it wants the same chocolate bar.

Yes, there are people like me who love Snickers, and then there are other people who just don't. It's not really about the Snickers, though. It's the same chocolate bar to the people who like it and who don't like it. It simply comes down to the individual taste of the person wanting the chocolate bar.

If she broke up with you, then you just weren't for her. Of course, there are countless reasons as to why she did it, and it's best after a break-up to exercise some self-awareness and reflect on the areas you can improve in. We all need to be open to growth and improvement, but all I can say is any future relationship you have will never reach its potential if you are stuck in a past rejection, too scared to commit yourself to love again.

THE ONE WHO NEVER SAID 'NO'
She let you get away with your shit until one day she just didn't. In fact, she barely had a voice in a relationship you controlled. Maybe she was the good girl who you treated like garbage, until she just couldn't put up with you a second longer. Or maybe she finally snapped, and things ended badly. She never said 'No' to you until one day she did – and it was over.

I've encountered many men in my journey who society would label as narcissists, to varying degrees. Personally, I believe this term is often overused and wrongly applied by people unqualified to make such a diagnosis, but there are definitely men with a very inflated sense of self-importance and entitlement, who treat their significant other with complete disregard. I've met men who refuse to ever hear their partner, or see anything beyond themselves or their own (often over-indulged) feelings.

Here's what I know to be true. Everyone has a breaking point. Absolutely everyone has a point where enough is enough. If you push someone hard enough, they will eventually snap. Her finally taking her power back, and saying 'No' to you, or 'Stop' or 'It's over', is actually the best thing for you. If you have been living in a warped version of reality, where no one can say 'No' to you, or you have to dominate her and every aspect of your life together, then treat her finally saying 'No' to you as a gift and a wake-up call. She has done you a huge favour. A healthy relationship is about an equal partnership of mutual respect. And it can be all too easy to slip into disrespecting someone who cannot say 'No' to you, without looking deeper. Regardless, whether she is assertive or passive (perhaps due to her own experiences of abuse), every woman deserves respect.

And just because she was a doormat for you for a period of time, that doesn't mean that anyone else will ever do this again for you. Unless you want to repeat this kind of relationship and find another victim to indulge you all over again, until they no longer can.

Brother, it's time to level up and recognise she is your equal – a woman who is a true match for you. A woman who knows her own worth enough to enforce boundaries, and who can say 'No', 'Stop' and 'That's enough!'

If you are trying your best to practise these old ways and beat her down into submission with controlling, abusive or manipulative behaviour, I want to tell you this: until you are willingly able to submit to a woman, and loan her the power to correct you, and call you out on your bad habits or dysfunctional behaviour, you will never ever reach your full potential as a man.

And I say this as a strong, opinionated male who, had I partnered with a woman who couldn't stand up to me, could very easily have been the one to walk all over her. My brothers and I often talk about how we are. We are strong – we've had to be to survive what we have – but we also need the kind of women who are confident to talk truth to bullshit, and call us out.

Having said this, how we behave shouldn't depend on how assertively our partner responds. How we behave and interact is our responsibility, not hers. From that point of view, then, my wahine toa has given me a gift and an opportunity. With her shining a light on my bullshit, I have had to lift my game and work out what is acceptable and what's not. That has helped me when I talk with Brothers whose partners might not be so forthright, shifting the focus and responsibility back to us. We are responsible for our actions and must accept accountability for our reactions.

It's not enjoyable when you have someone stand up to you, and challenge you. No one likes it at first. I've had to tell myself over the years that this woman challenging me isn't really challenging *me* - Matt Brown - as such, but rather some unhealthy thinking, warped ideas or misguided beliefs that I have learnt from living in abuse and dysfunction.

'Not everyone is worthy of our trust, and that is honestly why it is so much better to start any new relationship slowly.'

Sarah comes from a place of genuine desire, of wanting the best for me, just as I do for her, so I have been convinced that she is on my side, and in my corner, and that it is safe for me to allow her to correct me. I trust her motives and have learnt to not take correction as a personal attack. Taking correction without taking offence requires me to humble myself. So many of us men are prisoners of our own pride. We treat our women like our enemies, or as a threat when, really, they just want to be our friend, and to help us progress past the stuff that is actually holding us back, keeping us stuck in our past. Our pride flares up and we start being in 'attack mode' because we feel threatened. We have to realise that (often subconsciously) we have equated being corrected with criticism, so anything that she says - even innocently - to challenge our external behaviour, we actually feel is challenging something internally - like our worth or sense of belonging, or intellect.

A good example was a conversation I witnessed once between a couple I didn't really know well. They were attending a get-together at a mutual friend's home. The group were talking about their various university experiences, and the woman in the relationship had joined in, sharing about a moment of her postgraduate experience. It had probably gone on no longer than five minutes when, out of nowhere, her partner (who had stayed silent throughout the conversation) suddenly said:

'University doesn't mean everything – dumb people graduate all the time!' It was so random and out-of-the-blue that everyone just kind of stopped awkwardly.

His partner – clearly embarrassed – tried to smooth over the conversation with: 'I know heaps of people like you who make it in life without going down the path of higher education, but there are different paths for us all.' He made a snide remark to her about how she thought she was better than him because she had graduated from university, and huffed out of the room. She apologised to everyone, grabbed her bag and followed him quickly, so I never knew what happened after that.

But watching that encounter reminded me what it looks like when we haven't done the work inside ourselves, so we know what to do when we are triggered. An innocent comment triggers a feeling in us that we don't like. In this case, the Brother obviously struggled with feeling stupid or inadequate, so when he perceived everyone around him to be better than him, his feelings inside were triggered so badly that a huge overreaction occurred. It didn't matter to him how he embarrassed his partner, or whoever else it was in front of, in that moment. All that mattered to him was to do something to make his feelings of stupidity or inadequacy go away. In this situation, it was to try to bring down those around him, and minimise their qualifications. Those observing him in this situation saw a grown man having a tantrum. I saw a little boy feeling stupid.

THE ONE YOU CAN'T SEEM TO BREAK UP WITH, BUT NEED TO
It's like we can't stop touching the stove, even when it's burning us.

The relationships that are on this vicious emotional rollercoaster show the highs and lows of an emotional addiction. When it's good – usually because of physical passion – it's crazy good, but when it's bad – it's bad! It's volatile, unpredictable and unstable. You truly bring out each other's darkness, highlighting all your insecurities, and there's regular, ongoing conflict between you. Those who aren't committed to regularly doing the shadow work and exploring their own inner darkness cannot truly be aware of all they are bringing to their relationship.

You practise very few boundaries, and any semblance of a healthy, functional relationship might start to feel a bit boring to those who are used to these relationships of constant drama and abuse. It gets to the point where you're not really sure what to do with a love that is respectful and kind, calm and safe, and doesn't require you to consistently make painful self-sacrifices. I've known people with the latter relationship, yet somehow they are always drawn back to the craziness of an ex-partner because of an undeniable bond that hasn't properly been addressed and broken.

If this is you – and you potentially have a 'trauma bond' to someone you aren't currently with – then understand that really letting go of someone might seem impossible but it *is* possible. Sometimes we can be so bonded by shared trauma in a past relationship that we've built an attachment that has lasted longer than the relationship. You can become so intertwined with them that you can't imagine a life without them in it.

In this kind of situation, I encourage you to finish your business with them, and get some closure, so you can put your relationship to rest once and for all.

This might look like:

1. **Apologising to them for anything you regret.** For example, the way you treated them might still be playing on your mind, and since your relationship has ended you have had time to think and understand better. If it's possible to own your part, then maybe you can meet up and do just that. If meeting up with them isn't possible, then writing a heartfelt letter they may never have to read, to get your words and intentions out, can be just as powerful.

2. **Thanking them.** This person may be attached to you because they were such a significant part of your journey, so acknowledge that, and thank them for that, either in a conversation if you are able (and if it's

appropriate), or in a letter that, again, they may not necessarily ever have to read. They helped you get to where you are but, while that's important and beautiful, you don't necessarily need to keep going with them along their path.

3. **Grieving their loss in your life.** Find a way to do this without harming your current relationship. Be real about the good and the not-so-good parts of your time together. Understand that not everyone is a lifetime relationship – most are for a season, or a reason. So, for whatever reason, their season with you has come to an end. Acknowledge that. Allow yourself to sit with the feelings that come up for you. Feel the sadness that it's ended. Regret the way it may have ended. Hold onto that joy you felt for that moment in time that you loved each other. Feel gratitude for all the lessons learnt, which have brought you to where you are now.

4. **Giving yourself time.** Significant relationships take time to heal. After sharing our hearts, bodies and lives with another, we've bonded with them. It takes time to heal from that. It takes time to grieve that. Time that we need to give ourselves before we rush to another, and attempt to feel better in their arms. A rebound relationship will never give us what adequate and thoughtful closure will.

Focusing your thoughts, your time and your attention on any ex is focusing on the past and what is gone. She - the woman currently in your life - is your present and your future. She is someone to commit to growing with, learning alongside, and being challenged by.

Be here now, Brother. That is where love - and all of life - lives.

We can apply what we have learnt from our past relationships to our present one, but have the wisdom to let go of what is not for you anymore. Find the courage to say goodbye.

Chapter eight

She is not auditioning for you

IMAGINE A JOB INTERVIEW that never ended.

Or even a probationary employment period that never quite moved on from you proving you should be there, and that you have what it takes to do your position well.

Enter into a relationship that never seems to get past this stage, and it's an endless period of time where you constantly have to prove your worth to the other person in the relationship. It's like they have this underlying question that they can't decide to make a clear-cut decision on.

'Do I want to be with you or not?'

We live in an age where nothing seems clearly or easily defined.

'What are we?'

This seems to be the question people who are 'seeing' people have to ask. They have repeated discussions about this with their friends, their colleagues and their Mothers. Are we together? Are we exclusive? I think so, but I don't know for sure, because we are just seeing how things go, and, right now, we are 'down for whatever'!

This isn't even something that is being said within weeks or months of meeting someone and dating them regularly. This is being said by people who are *years in* – by people living together, and even by people with children together!

What does 'down for whatever' really even mean? How does that work for a relationship? How do you go about the task of building trust or developing intimacy with this concept? What happens when the feelings one person has for the other inevitably develop? It's like you want the closeness and benefits of what a relationship offers, and having someone to depend on, without any of the commitment that a functional, healthy, reciprocal relationship asks for.

I meet so many guys who aren't sure. They have one foot in the bed and one foot out the door. Recently, I asked a client, Phil, while I was blading him up after giving him his weekly fade, if he was in or out with a girl he had been 'seeing' for well over a year.

He kind of shrugged and said: 'I haven't decided.'

'What are you waiting on from her to decide?' I asked.

'I don't actually know,' he said. 'I do like her, and we get along well, but I guess I don't know for sure if she's it for me. I mean, what if someone hotter came along?'

And that was it, folks. He was waiting for someone hotter.

He was essentially keeping this girl of his – who he told me he liked (and probably told her he loved) – auditioning for him for over a year, because he hadn't decided if she was hot enough for him.

I kid you not: these conversations are had in barber's chairs all over the world, without doubt, every other day. That's the beauty of being a barber – you hear it all! Absolutely nothing shocks me now.

'What if she finds someone hotter, and moves on from you, Bro? And then you realise she's the girl of your dreams and you've missed your chance to seal the deal because you kept her in the audition phase for too long, and she then gets signed by someone else who sees her beauty on day one?'

He laughed. 'Won't happen, Bro. Treat her mean to keep her keen. Trust me, she loves me.'

Oh, I was sure she did – as the many before her did. He is an attractive, confident guy, with a good personal training business. But why? Why did she love a man who had her auditioning for a place in his life, and waiting for him to deem her 'hot enough' to commit to?

I appreciated his honesty, but I felt sad in that moment. Was this the future for my daughters? Is this behaviour just accepted now? In this era of fighting for women's equality were there really women just sitting around for a year, waiting for guys like him – who weren't sure if they even wanted them – to pick them?

I started asking around and, unfortunately, I found an epidemic of men who refused to be 'all in'. This audition phase was like an actual, recognised part of life now:

1. Meet a girl.

2. Date her.

3. Decide you like her enough to say you are 'seeing her' and string her along on multiple dates to get her interested.

4. Now this is where people are getting stuck: audition her. Keep her in this phase. Don't make anything too official, *but* give her enough incentive to keep her in this zone, as long as she'll stay there. Make her feel like you *are* interested, *but* there's just something you aren't sure of – so she keeps working hard to prove herself, shows you her unconditional love, her loyalty, her brilliant culinary skills, her yoga expertise in bed. You still aren't sure, so you keep her working hard and she keeps on auditioning. It never seems to end until she finally threatens that it *is* the end. That's when you do some pseudo-connection shit like a teary 'I love you', followed by you sharing the story of previously getting your heart broken, or being abandoned and feeling scared by these feelings, and could she please now just bear with you as you navigate

your way *slowly* through these feelings. She agrees, and you have passionate sex, and she's feeling closer to you than *ever*. But it never really progresses from there. The navigation you spoke of? The boat never really leaves the dock!

5. Officially (and finally!) be 'all in' in a committed relationship, which – *yes* – means everyone knows you are together. You're even official on social media now.

6. Pop the question and get engaged. If you like it, you better put a ring on it!

7. Seal the deal. You have decided you are 'all in' forever, so you make her your *wife!*

THERE SEEMS TO BE a lot less of phases 5, 6 and 7 if I'm to be honest.

I'm finding men who want the best of both worlds – they say they want the freedom of being single, but the comfort of having a relationship.

These are men who want to keep their options wide open. Because, like Phil, they think that a better girl (whatever that means) might come along. Men who may technically be even living with her, but wouldn't actually say they were, so they'd keep some stuff somewhere else, and on Saturday nights go out on a bender with the boys and not have to go home to her because – you guessed it – they don't really live there, even though they spend most of the week with her.

Men who Father children with her, but he can't even commit to his children, and doesn't fully live with them either.

Where did this lack of commitment come from? Are we the generation known for not committing to anything or anyone properly?

When did we suddenly think it was okay to string someone along for extended periods of time? I think it's down to the sheer number of options available to us at the literal touch of a button.

Look at the world of dating apps. Suddenly you have thousands of available people in your area, lined up, ready for selection. You don't have to do much to select them either - you're at home, you swipe left or right depending on your mood for the day. You see instantly if they are 'down for whatever', too. You flick through a quick message to meet up and - here is where my mind boggles - one of my former clients tells me he meets girls from his car.

You heard me.

He tells them to meet him in a carpark so he can see if he even wants to bother to grab a drink.

Yep, it's an audition for a drink.

I couldn't believe it, but he said he always does it - and tells me that girls are apparently 'fine' with it. Are they really? Or are so many getting duped into thinking there is no alternative? Why would a woman be vulnerable and put herself out there if he's not willing to meet her past the carpark?

I think back to how dating or courtship worked only a few generations ago, when you met people in the vicinity of where you were in life. Generally it was confined to your city, or even specifically to your village or neighbourhood. You typically met through your school, your church, a community group, or where you worked. There were, obviously, a limited number of people available to you in your area at any given time who were of a suitable age, and not already taken.

You put your best foot forward and gave it some effort. If you liked what you saw, you asked her out, and - because there weren't a thousand other girls ready and waiting in your pocket to swipe right to - you actually gave it a good go. If you liked her, you told her, then you dated her, and then after an appropriate courtship period you decided whether she was the one, and if she was you asked her to marry you and then you got married.

It does seem simpler, doesn't it?

Of course, I understand this period of time was not without its challenges. Couples still had their problems then - there's no era in history when people didn't have relationship conflict - but does the seemingly unlimited immediate access we have now to so much choice actually help us to live the life that most people say they want?

I don't think so.

I don't think I have met a single person who doesn't on some level want to love and to be loved. The thing is, to attain this love you say you want you must actually be 'all in' – not in that limbo phase of a never-ending audition.

Ask any performer: auditioning is exhausting. You're always putting your best face forward, always 'on' to perform. There's never any time to relax or just be 'you', because you never know which 'you' is wanted. Imagine living like that full-time. Imagine that this is how your girlfriend, or partner, is living, simply because you can't make a decision – to commit, or quit.

And don't mistake what I'm saying to mean that you should be moving in with her the first week you meet. There's wisdom in dating someone and actually finding out who they are, and what they are about, but this period seems to get so unnecessarily prolonged, in my opinion.

When I say 'all in', I mean decided and committed that love with this girl is essentially worth the risk of heartbreak.

Ouch. Here we have it.

To attain any kind of real-deal love you could potentially get hurt.

There's nothing you can do to avoid this, I'm afraid. To truly be connected to her, and have a love where you are fully known and fully seen, means you have to decide to step forward and have both feet in. I know to some of you this sounds scary. It is.

But I promise you, it's worth it! Emotional intimacy is worth every bit of the vulnerability required to achieve it. To stay in that 'audition phase' will not ever give you what you want. No risk – no reward.

When I think back to how my relationship began with Sarah, I think back to when I decided I was 'all in'.

We had been best friends for four years. For three of those years we didn't live in the same city, and part of the time we weren't even in the same country, as she had moved to the beautiful island of Rarotonga in the Cook Islands. We stayed in touch via phone calls and online. It was strictly a platonic friendship for that time. There were no blurred lines or physical intimacy of any kind. In the fourth year of our friendship she moved cities to where I lived in Christchurch, New Zealand.

Sarah agreed to come for one year to help me grow my business, bringing along her daughter, who was then only nine years old. At the time I was still working from the tin shed where I started my barbering, before I moved into the larger barbershop that I still have now.

I appreciated her help, and her time, because she could have been working anywhere, for anyone, and here she was - helping a guy in a tin shed. But it was her belief in me - and her belief in and support of my work in connecting with the men in my hood way back then - that cemented the foundation of everything we do today.

When she arrived at the start of 2013, it was post the tragic 2011 earthquake that had completely devastated our city, so we were in the process of rebuilding across the city. Accommodation was scarce, so she lived with my older sister and her family. I'll never forget that. My wife has always been a very independent, self-sufficient person since she left home as a 15-year-old, so to live with my family just so she could help me grow my business truly meant so much to me.

That year I saw her for real.

I saw Sarah's genuine love for people who many overlook in our society - the vulnerable, the minorities, the traumatised. I saw her fierce love for her daughter, Oceana. She wasn't a Mother who let anything - or anyone - slide around her. She was protective of her daughter's body, mind and spirit - and so mindful of everything in Oceana's world. I deeply admired that about her because, as a child, I hadn't felt protected at all. She was everything I felt a parent should be.

I saw her tender heart, I knew that she was on her own journey of healing from the tremendous rejection and abandonment she had faced from the very start of her life, but she had the courage and determination to push through. I saw her work ethic - no one worked harder in the room than Sarah. She loved to make plans for the business, then set goals and find ways to accomplish them. She was always solutions-based – nothing was ever a problem, including not having any money to make our dreams a reality! She always found a way, and was creative, focused and ambitious in how she achieved those goals.

I saw Sarah's love for me. She was the very best friend I have ever had in all my life. Honest. Loyal. Empathetic. Kind. Inspiring. She inspired me to be kinder, braver and more generous. She kept her word, and knew what I needed: for her to show up for me. She could handle the truth of who I was. I didn't have to be anyone other than who I was with her. How liberating and refreshing.

A year passed. It was now the start of 2014. We had accomplished so much. I had left my tin barber shed, and we had worked hard to raise the money needed to set up my dream barbershop. I had even left the country for the first time, and travelled around the USA for two months with her and my other best friend, Josh, visiting barbershops from Las Vegas to New York City, soaking up that barbershop culture the USA is so renowned for.

When Sarah went on a date one evening in January and I babysat Oceana, I didn't like this feeling I was starting to feel. I knew I didn't want her to date anyone else. But here I was, scared shitless. Like I mentioned earlier, I had told myself – and her throughout our entire friendship – that I was called and destined for celibacy. Yep, I was to live the life of a monk. By choice.

Of course, knowing what I know now, it was just my way of protecting myself – of staying hidden. As someone who had been sexually violated on numerous occasions throughout my childhood and adolescent years, I had decided that sex with a partner just wasn't for me. So I shut that part of myself down, in an effort to protect what had been defiled. Most of us who have felt exposed, violated or unprotected as children do this in various ways. It's our natural way of coping.

So, in this moment, these budding, unfamiliar feelings for her were directly the opposite to what I had convinced myself of for years. And they were inviting me to risk everything.

I had a choice – we always do. I could choose to accept this invitation to feel something new with her, or I could shut these blossoming feelings down and live in a way my heart no longer wanted to live. I was safe here, wasn't I? Did I really want to risk everything I knew for the possibility of love, or should I just keep on clinging to the safety of what I thought I knew?

I thought long and hard. It was the biggest decision of my life. I knew Sarah. She had shown herself to me these past four years. I saw who she really was. I saw her strengths and her weaknesses. I knew that to take her on was to also take on her daughter and to be a Father to her, too. Did I have what it took when I was barely fathered myself? All my inadequacies popped up to the surface. I had struggled with my identity and sexuality after the abuse, I had struggled with a pornography addiction, I had never even had consensual intercourse with anyone – so could I really do this with her?

Somewhere deep within, I found this seed of courage. And a seed is all we need to plant a forest.

What does love do? I asked myself. Love finds a way. Love liberates our fears. Love heals our hurt. Love sets us free to be the best version of ourselves. **Love makes all things possible.**

So on the evening of 13 January 2014, I told Sarah that I loved her as more than just a friend. I told Sarah that I didn't just want to date her, but that I planned to marry her. I wanted Oceana to be my daughter – not my stepdaughter, because I don't believe in that term – but my daughter. I told her I had weighed it all up, and here I was asking her to say 'Yes' to me.

Because I saw her, I knew her, and I loved her in a way I had never loved anyone before. I wanted my life, however that looked, and whatever it brought, with them both by my side.

I remember Sarah looked at me with tear-filled eyes.

'Are you sure?' she asked.

'Yes,' I said. 'So sure.'

I had never been more sure about anything else in my entire life.

From that one decision – to choose love with her that January night – came the entire life that I had dreamt of as a kid in the hood, an alternative to where home was a battleground and abuse was normal. Where there was no food, but plenty of beatings. Where alcohol made every situation worse, and anyone had unlimited access to us children in our own home. I would often lie awake at night and dream with my little brother Paul about what our life would one day be like, in this alternative world.

I dreamt of love like a nineties R&B love song. I dreamt of lots of laughter and delicious meals like I had seen on TV shows, where families sat around together and talked. I dreamt of holidays with my children, and watching them grow up with my soulmate and my best friend.

Saying 'Yes' to love when I was scared was like opening the door to the life I really wanted, but had never thought was actually possible for me.

I'm here to tell you: it *is* possible, Brother.

My life shows you it was possible for me then.

It is possible for you now.

It is always possible, if we have the courage to do something different.

Won't you take the courage inside of yourself to say 'Yes' to love, and 'Yes' to opening the door on the life you really want?

Because everything you want is right there on the other side of the door. That door is called vulnerability, and it's inviting you to love.

Consider the following . . .

- What are you looking for in a life partner?

- What do you have to offer this potential partner? Are you these things, too?

- Do you have any subconscious beliefs about relationships that aren't helpful to the relationship you are in now? For example, beliefs that have nothing to do with her and everything to do with a past experience that you need to do some work on to heal from.

- How long will you let a relationship drift on before you discuss what your next steps will be together?

Chapter nine

She is not your porn star

SHE IS NOT YOUR PORN STAR, your stripper, prostitute or escort - in fact, she is not your *paid* sex worker at all, so she doesn't *owe* you anything.

Can reality ever compete with a fantasy?

Brothers, we need to tell ourselves the truth about sex workers. They are paid to do a job, and that is to please you for the time you have paid for. You are deluding yourself if you believe anything else, and if they are good at their job then I can genuinely see why the confusion exists. And while I acknowledge sex workers as working in a legitimate industry that there is a huge demand for, I personally do not believe that using sex workers has any place in my own committed, monogamous relationship. In our marriage we seek sexual intimacy in a number of different ways with each other.

A male friend of mine is addicted to pornography and has been for years. It transitioned from watching countless hours of pornography daily to frequenting brothels and having sex with prostitutes, because it eventually got to the point where he wanted the real thing. At one point his delusion was so great that he really believed that he was 'the exception'. He almost bragged about being the one that the girls enjoyed having sex with – with them telling him 'he was different from other clients – cleaner, more attractive, etc'. And he would lap up their words and feed his ego with them, believing that they looked forward to his visits. This is the same guy who had never been in any functional, committed relationship with a woman, and he was by then in his mid-thirties.

Porn stars are X-rated movie actors who film sexual fantasies – mostly for the benefit of heterosexual men – so their videos can generate huge revenue for those producing them. Sadly, only a tiny percentage of the huge revenue created in the billion-dollar online mainstream pornography industry actually goes to the actors starring in those videos. The porn stars themselves are not the ones making the biggest cut in this lucrative industry.

In fact, there are millions of women and children trafficked into the porn industry from all over the world who are not even making a single dollar. They are being exploited, and those of us who are watching free pornography need to tell ourselves there is a very high chance that what we are consuming for our own gratification and enjoyment is very likely the rape and exploitation of a young person.

The psychological effects on young men growing up in this age of instant sexual gratification at their fingertips is that many men (and boys) have a skewed sense of relationships, consent and intimacy. They believe women are always ready to have sex at any moment, and will sexually please them in any way possible, including degrading herself. It portrays women as disposable – it's easy to 'tap and run'. Violence and pornography are also inextricably connected, with studies proving a huge increase in verbal and physical aggression from those consuming pornography regularly.

This doesn't surprise me in the slightest, as the majority of the messaging in free mainstream pornography is that coercing, disrespecting, and physically and verbally abusing women is acceptable. You can't watch that daily and *not* have it affect how you treat women, and what you believe about them, because we become what we consume.

Pornography generally portrays men as being powerful and in control, while women are shown to be submissive and obedient, doing whatever the men desire and demand.

To put it bluntly, so much of what is considered mainstream, easily accessible pornography is basically women being beaten up and raped while smiling.

Watching hours and hours of submissive women being dehumanised makes it seem normal, but it also sets us up to believe that our own relationships don't have to be equal in power, and that varying degrees of verbal and physical abuse against women are acceptable.

However, there is a school of thought that some pornography can be seen as 'ethical', and there are female content-creators who attempt to create porn that models consensual, loving, caring relationships. I know there are also numerous platforms where women feel empowered to create their own sexual content and charge money directly from consumers, therefore being able to create revenue fairly on their own terms. I want to be very clear that pornography like this is not the type of pornography that I encountered growing up.

My first encounter with pornography was at home, with my parents watching videos in the lounge while having sex in front of us. My younger brother recalls this being one of his first memories at three years old, and he can still remember vividly the details of the video, including a blue shoe that featured in it.

Because pornography was a 'normal' part of our childhood, it set us all up for exposure to sexual abuse and incest. At the time it was also culturally taboo to talk about sex in a healthy, functional way, so we were all sexually awoken long before we were emotionally ready to deal with sex, with no one to guide us down a tricky path we weren't ready to go down.

At eight years old I distinctly recall watching my Father's stash of porn videos with my older sister and my younger brother while my parents were at work, and by the age of 13 I was secretly watching it on a computer in the art room at school. It was in a separate room, and my teacher trusted me in that space outside of class hours because I was also a keen artist. This would occur once or twice a fortnight, and continued right through high school.

I have never watched pornography with anyone else, as I did feel a sense of shame about it, but there were occasions when boys would bring magazines along to school, inevitably from their Father's stash, and some would even sell individually ripped-out pages for a dollar.

As I got older I would watch porn secretly from an internet café, choosing my position and computer carefully in a corner, so I wouldn't be caught out. In my early twenties I bought my first smartphone, which suddenly meant unlimited access and options wherever I was.

At the height of my addiction I was binge-watching porn about three times a day. I did kind of want to quit, in theory, but only for the religious reasons drilled into us as Polynesian teens attending church: that sex was forbidden before marriage. We were repeatedly told that all lust was sinful and that Hell was a very real place for sinners. None of this did anything practical to help a porn-addicted young man who had already been sexually abused from a young age, and who was struggling with the onset of raging adolescent hormones while telling himself he should be celibate.

I kept watching and felt guilty, so I would stop myself from watching for short periods of time, before inevitably succumbing to temptation and binge-watching again on my phone. At the time I didn't understand that I was wiring my brain to want to watch porn more often – and that my porn addiction was comparable to a substance addiction, like smoking or taking drugs. Watching it fired up pleasure centres in my brain, and every fix demanded more watching.

Real change in this area only took place when I met Sarah. She humanised the women I had previously just considered as 'porn stars'. At the time she was working for an aid and development agency, and one of her big passions was raising awareness and funds to fight the evil that is human trafficking. The agency she worked at had a partnership with International Justice Mission, a charity that is one of the largest anti-slavery organisations in the world.

A big part of their work highlights sex trafficking – when a woman or child is forced into commercial sexual exploitation for profit. Victims are held against their will, and forced into brothels or similar places, to be sold over and over again to paying clients. Some are forced into the porn industry, where they are often drugged and raped repeatedly, or forced into cyber sex-trafficking, where they are filmed being abused at the direction of the paying client over a webcam. This sadly occurs in countries and communities all over the world.

For Sarah, these people were not nameless statistics, but real people who were someone's daughters and sons. She showed me countless stories of women who had left the porn industry and were brave enough to share their stories. Many had come into the industry as children or young women. Some also came from abuse backgrounds similar to mine, and their desperation and pain were exploited by those porn-film producers. Most were trying to escape a less-than-desirable life, and this may have seemed like a way out.

'We become what we consume.'

In their stories and interviews, however, it became clear that it was far from an 'easy life', and the picture they painted behind the scenes was truly hell, where the only way of coping with the long hours of physical and sexual exploitation and violence was to attempt to blank out or numb their experiences with drug use. Many workers in the industry were drugged-up and addicted just so they could cope, and most of their earnings were spent feeding their addictions.

Humanising the people on my screen – who I had never considered before – meant that it just wasn't the same to watch anymore, and I seriously tried to stop. So many men I know who watch pornography regularly admit that they wouldn't be comfortable watching someone raped directly in front of them – yet why is it so different via a screen?

Research shows that children these days are exposed to pornography often around the age of eight – and it can be down to something as innocent as searching for something online that brings a pornographic image onto their screens. Often children are unsure if they can raise this kind of topic with their parents, because so many parents seem to want to skip the 'facts of life' sex discussion, relying on schools to tell their kids about puberty and the body. And shame thrives on secrecy, silence and judgement.

Exposure to violent pornography at a young age can set children up to try out what they see on the screen with their friends; impact their wellbeing; skew their ideas about healthy sexual relationships, gender equality and consent; and normalise early sexual behaviour. It can lead to young people sending each other sexually explicit images via smartphones or digital devices, which can lead to potential for blackmail and cyberbullying. Children start believing that the sexual practices they see on screen are what happen in real-life relationships.

BY THE TIME I was sitting across from a well-known and highly skilled therapist, I was ready to change – by any means possible. Sarah sat next to me in support.

I was nervous, as I wasn't sure what to expect, but I decided I would lay it all out to him because I was so tired of hiding. I knew without a doubt that my only chance of ever truly beating this addiction was complete transparency, which meant bringing everything hidden and shameful to the light.

As a boy who was so used to being physically exposed from such a young age, I had to really get my head around transparency. I came to realise that transparency and exposure were completely different, because transparency was on my terms, in the safety of a relationship I trusted, whereas exposure was not on my terms, and was done with people I couldn't trust.

My therapist David was incredible. He listened intently, and immediately gave me some truthful insights, which I still remember to this day, and will share with you here. For a long time after this session I would take out my coaching sheet and re-read it daily, so I could basically rewire my unhealthy thinking by applying the truth.

If you struggle with an addiction to pornography, too, I invite you to use the tools I found so helpful at the time. I also recommend that you seek professional help if you are struggling. We can't always try to fix this alone – there are times when we need professional expertise, and it's not weak or shameful to ask for help.

Some of the truthful insights David gave me into my pornography addiction were:

- Living a double life will *never* work, and pornography will never make my life better.

- Pornography is repetitive and boring. There is nothing really new to see, and it just feeds the desire to see more shocking images. Where will watching this pornography end up for me?

- I can resist the desire to watch it. The desire itself is not permanent, it is only temporary and it won't last long if I keep resisting it.

- I will stop consuming pornography while I have the power to do so, and before I become a dirty old man, which is not who I want to be.

- With every resistance to watching pornography, the desire will lose some of its grip. It won't always be this hard.

- Doing anything in secret is an illusion. There is no 'in secret', as it will all be made known eventually.

- The desire is *within* me because of my original awakening, but it is not *of* me unless I continue to indulge it.

- Pornography separates sex from communication, loyalty, love and affection, and thereby spoils the natural excitement, producing boredom instead.

- Pornography removes boundaries and the dignity of others. Watching someone being raped on a screen is no different in principle to watching it in my lounge for my own pleasure.

- Erotic desire escalates. What do I need to see next in its ever-increasing need for indulgence and satisfaction?

- Pornography is not victimless. It exists to the detriment of the porn stars themselves.

I still have the sheet that he wrote out for me to refer to after our session together. It was dated 9 July 2014. I am proud to write that I have not watched any pornography since that date. That's literally years of being clean from an addiction that had been part of my life since I was a young boy.

Make no mistake, there have been moments over the years where the temptation or urge has come over me. But I am now able to coach myself through it, without giving in. The longer it has been, the less often the desires have come. Initially, I read those coaching truths daily, and repeated them to myself constantly. There was no other option for me – I knew who I didn't want to be, and I was committed to doing whatever was necessary to find a solution to be free from the detrimental effects of pornography.

I'LL NEVER FORGET SEEING an interview with a favourite gospel singer of mine, where he revealed his secret porn addiction. What sticks in my mind is the response of his wife in that interview, talking about how having sex with him ended up making *her* feel dirty. This was because of the demands and requests he made of her. He wanted her to re-enact the porn he was consuming on a regular basis.

There is no way a real-life woman can ever compete with someone acting and playing the part of turning us on, on demand. A real-life woman has her own needs and emotions, and doesn't exist solely to please us when we want them to.

Sex and intimacy, in my experience, are better enjoyed in a loving, mutually respectful relationship, where both people get their needs and desires met. When I think of sexual intimacy with my wife, having an orgasm is literally only 1% of it, because I believe intimacy is really about truth.

So many people equate intimacy with sex. But when you realise you can tell someone your whole truth – when you can really show yourself to them, and you stand in front of them with nothing to hide, and their response is 'You're safe with me' – that's intimacy.

Intimacy: Into – Me – See.

She is not my porn star, or a sex worker providing me with an easy cheap 'fix', but, rather, she is my lover, my equal, and my safe place to be vulnerable enough to show her all of me . . . *my beloved*.

And until we are really prepared to see women as our equals, we will justify their degradation in multiple ways every day. We can excuse the locker-room talk, the barbershop banter, and the way that 'she' can be constantly belittled and humiliated – called a bitch, a slut or a ho. We can even make her think she *likes* to be referred to by these names, so much so that she now refers to herself as this. We can ignore the constant dehumanisation in song lyrics that we all like and know, and sing along with because there is nothing wrong, right? It's just a catchy beat and it's got a good vibe.

It's an ongoing conflict.

I grew up in the era of nineties hip-hop, and I'm a huge fan of Tupac Shakur. To me, he is a symbol of resistance, and I genuinely view him as not only the greatest rapper of all time, a prophet and a poet – but also as a Father figure of sorts to many of us from a generation of absent Fathers. The man who first taught me how to express pain with words, and inspired me to have the courage to own my own story, as excruciating as it was.

It's always been a complex conflict within me – to be both a huge hip-hop fan and consumer, but also be someone who would view himself as a feminist – a man who wants the same opportunities, access and treatment for my daughters as I want for my son. With many rap lyrics, these two parts of myself seem incompatible, as so much of the hip-hop genre I grew up with is filled with misogyny.

What even *is* misogyny? At its core it is a hatred or mistrust of women. It is a prejudice against women in a culture that promotes men above women, and stereotypes women's roles, language and behaviour, and enforces sexism. It is something that has existed throughout history, alongside patriarchy – which is a social system where men hold most of the power, operate in most of the leadership roles, and hold a position of control over women and children. Patriarchy automatically assumes that men are the head of the household, the company or the political system.

'Pornography is not victimless.'

My view is that you can appreciate the art form of rap and hip-hop, while also understanding that it is a by-product of its time. It is an audio representation of the cultural, political and historical climate that the rapper grew up in. It is a landscape that shows us all so clearly the way many men think about, communicate about, and engage with, women.

Like many rappers of the 'gangsta rap' genre of hip-hop, Tupac was a young African-American male, born in Harlem, New York, who moved to Baltimore and later to California. He grew up surrounded by huge inequality and poverty and a short supply of adequate welfare, social services, street safety and education. In this environment, these brutal dynamics are a breeding ground for sexism's most brutal manifestations: domestic violence, sexual abuse and exploitation, and rape.

With astronomical numbers of Fathers from his generation incarcerated – a direct result of slavery and racism – so many boys like Tupac grew up in unstable homes with absent or addicted parents. Then, longing for belonging and connection in the inner-city slums they lived in (known as the Projects or government housing blocks), this support was then found in gangs, the drug trade, physical or sexual violence, and in hip-hop culture.

So although Tupac was part of reinforcing the sexism that is rife throughout hip-hop's gangsta rap culture, with his derogatory references to 'bitches', many of his songs also communicated messages of love and deep respect. He shared through his verses how he viewed and felt a deep love for women, too, being raised by a strong single Mother alongside his Sister. Tracks like his 1991 hit 'Brenda's Got a Baby' or his 1995 track for his Mother, 'Dear Mama', show the heart of the man who thought and cared deeply.

On his first album to go platinum, the 1993 hit *Strictly 4 my N.I.G.G.A.Z.*, Tupac used his voice to encourage women in the struggle he saw first-hand in his world. With my favourite track of his, 'Keep Ya Head Up', Tupac's clear message is that he cares for these women. He reinforces their self-worth, and he speaks truth to everyone's existence – we wouldn't be here if it wasn't for women. His lyrics can go from calling her 'Bitch' to 'Sista', but he also shows that he understands the essential role women play in our lives, and the respect we need to show them if we are to continue on.

It makes me question myself, too. Am I, Matt Brown, in 2021, really that different from a nineties gangsta rapper? Have my own roots in patriarchal masculinity ever really been completely challenged?

Remember, the subconscious thoughts we have that are yet to be challenged are the most powerful until we challenge or interrogate them. Ask yourself these questions:

- Do you subconsciously think women are inferior to you?

- Do you allow your own thinking about and ideas of women to evolve?

- As you know and understand better, do you *do* better in every area of your life?

- Do you speak up for women's systematic oppression in almost every area of life – from workplaces to churches to brothels?

- How do you react when you hear powerful men in the most powerful positions in the world say things like, 'Grab 'em by the pussy. You can do anything.'

American feminist writer bell hooks says: 'The power of the patriarchy has been to make maleness feared and to make men believe that it is better to be feared than to be loved. Whether they can confess this or not, men know that just is not true.'

It is not true, yet in the culture of mainstream pornography, fear is the over-riding theme that continues to be communicated, so that the power over and control of women can continue. How can she ever rise when he has her naked on the ground, choking her while simultaneously squirting semen on her face? How can she rise while men take pleasure in her defilement? How can we rise when this image still excites so many of us?

bell hooks also says: 'Imagine how much easier it would be for us, to learn how to love if we began with a shared definition.'

A shared definition.

A collaboration.

A partnership.

A world where her equality would not threaten us, but rather thrill us.

Where she could be everything *she* wanted, and we would celebrate her success, her evolution and her ascension, because we would see it as *our* success – our evolution and our ascension as a collective race of people.

Brothers, are we willing to evolve?

Chapter ten

She is not your prison

THE QUESTION IS: Who or what are you really trying to escape from?

She is not your prison guard or your jailer, yet so many of us men treat her as something we have to escape from.

I have had countless conversations with men who act like their life and world with their partner and children are something they need to break free from on a regular basis.

Like they somehow deserve a 'free pass' on the weekends to do whatever they want, with no regard whatsoever to her needs, or the needs of those dependent on them. After 'an exhausting week at work' they now deserve all the time they need to themselves to unwind. Like she and their children are a prison of life they really don't want, and didn't sign up for.

Sometimes it comes across that the grown-ass man in front of me is actually a petulant child who doesn't want to grow up and be an adult.

Never mind that she is also tired after working in a job outside the home all week, or having looked after children at home –

which is, in my experience, more exhausting than working a paid job. Never mind that she and your children (if you have them) have probably looked forward to time with you all week, but now you'd rather do anything but be present with them.

I'm not suggesting we don't all deserve and need time to ourselves, but yet again *your* time alone cannot come at the expense of *her* time for herself that she also deserves. I'd like to think that the over-riding message of this book is for you to consider her feelings, and realise that your healing and enjoyment in life cannot come at the expense of hers. In fact, her feelings should be just as important as your feelings when it comes to any decisions you make.

Moderation and negotiation are essential skills to practise in most things, and they're something that a functional relationship requires. If you want to plan a big Friday night out with the boys after work, then planning and discussing that with her *prior* to the day is only fair. If you want to spend all day on Saturday playing sports with your friends, then, again, this can be discussed. There is a vast difference between activities used to escape or avoid your life, and activities used for recreation and enjoyment. Is it fair that Dad opts out of family life every damn weekend just to blow off some steam?

I'm going to be straight-up here and tell you – man-to-man – that you don't get to 'opt out' of your relationship and run away from family life whenever you feel like it. It's time to grow up and realise that family life, or a committed relationship, like anything, comes with highs and lows. And how you ride out both of these determines the quality of life not only for yourself, but what you subsequently create for (and with) your family.

Yes, there are those awesome times together. For example, when you enjoy a nice family dinner and the kids aren't fighting, or when you just stand there in awe of the little humans you have both created who are growing up so fast right in front of you.

There are exciting times together, like being able to go on a family holiday that you've saved up for and looked forward to. There are stressful times together, when there is a loss of income, or an unexpected bill that puts financial pressure on you as a couple, which sometimes means you can't provide for your children in quite the way you'd want to.

There are sad moments when a sickness or loss comes to you, and the grief you have to experience together as a family is immeasurable.

And then there is the boring monotony that sometimes is daily life. When it seems as though you are running on a treadmill of working, cooking, raising kids, sleeping, and repeating that for the longest period with very little excitement. These moments seem to occur more often than not, and I've learned to find joy in the small things, and truly enjoy those parts of life, because strangely enough they are the moments that mean the most.

'Who or what are you really trying to escape from?'

There's nothing I enjoy more than a home-cooked meal with my people. I appreciate the smell of my wife's homemade bread or eating the boil-up soup she makes. I count myself blessed with the effort she makes for our family. I look forward to chats with my son at bedtime, and making up crazy bedtime stories where he is the superhero fighting a giant T-Rex to save his baby sister. I love holding my little baby girl, and just snuggling her close, as I know she won't be this small for long. I enjoy taking my teenage daughter out for one-on-one Dad and daughter time. Things as simple as waking up a bit earlier than usual so we can drive to McDonald's and eat breakfast together, just the two of us, before work and school – that's something we both look forward to all week. Sarah and I don't always have access to babysitters, so sometimes a date just means snuggling up on the couch with a new Netflix show and some snacks. These moments are not particularly glamorous, exciting or newsworthy, but they are affordable little things we can find enjoyment in daily.

We can afford to save for a good family holiday every couple of years, but we do our best in between these holidays to get out of town for even a day, or a weekend, with our family for mini adventures, so we try to have little things we can look forward to. Even just planning to do inexpensive activities around the city we live in is fun, and I look forward to my days off so that I can spend my time with my favourite people.

We create the life we want, and if you feel you are living in a prison, then you need to take responsibility for the prison that you have created. Your life can be as fun or even as miserable as you want. I suggest if you are stuck in the mentality of wanting to party every weekend and escape the people you probably do really want to spend the bulk of your time with, then you need to reassess your life and your priorities.

I love a night with my Brothers or close friends. I love to enjoy a glass of good whisky and some lively man-to-man conversation. Is it fair that I do this every weekend after my wife has had the kids all week while I have been at work? Hell no! So I always run the idea past Sarah to check that we don't have anything else planned first, and that she's feeling okay with not having me around for an evening. She returns the courtesy if she wants to pop out for dinner or a movie with her friends and Sisters. It's not us asking for permission from each other, either – it's healthy to do things away from each other – but it's considerate to check in with your partner when making alternative plans for a time you'd otherwise be together.

Right now we have two young children (along with a teenager), which inevitably means that sleep is sometimes scarce, and after a long week with very little sleep it's just not cool to leave my wife to handle the kids alone, exhausted, while I party with my friends. During many nights of exhaustion we have both looked at each other and said 'There is no one I'd rather do this life with than you!'

And the 'prison' of child-rearing and work doesn't seem like a prison when you are in it together with your best friend.

IF YOU ARE SOMEONE who sees your family life or relationship as a prison, then ask yourself why, and **what exactly do you**

positively contribute to your life together to make it enjoyable?

I asked these exact questions to a client I've been cutting for the past few years. Will had a committed and loyal wife, but following the birth of their child he started going out more than ever. He had just started a reasonably good business, just bought a house, and it was like an instant change. Every weekend he started drinking, partying on Friday with friends until Saturday morning, when he would spend the day asleep, then he would wake up and repeat it again on Saturday night. Sunday was again spent sleeping the day away in recovery.

This went on for months until one day, in desperation, she told him to pack up his stuff and move to his single friend's bachelor pad permanently. At first he seemed elated. He told me he felt free and was having fun - the 'time of his life' he said. Frequent visits to strip clubs meant he was also now casually sleeping around with girls younger than his wife.

I cut his hair weekly, and would always ask him how he was doing. My role as a barber is mostly to listen, and I only ever offer advice when it's asked for.

One day, months down the track, he admitted to me he wasn't actually that happy. He missed his wife, and he felt he was now missing all the milestones of his growing baby.

'Isn't this what you wanted, though?' I asked him quietly, as I was lining him up. Looking at him in the mirror, I could see he was tired.

'I thought it was,' he admitted, 'but it doesn't feel like freedom anymore. I think I've sabotaged what I really do want.'

I asked him what freedom looked like to him, and why he had thought his home life was a prison of sorts. His response was not too different from what other men have confided in me.

Home life seemed boring, monotonous, and it felt like everything now revolved around their small child. They had very little family support, and their baby had some health issues, which meant sleep was rare as their child was up most nights with stomach pains. There was less time for him and less attention from her.

He felt disappointed in himself for not providing the quality of life he imagined he'd have by now, and felt pressure as the sole provider with his wife now being on maternity leave. There was less money for the fun things they had once enjoyed together, and he felt that after being the only one to 'work a job' all week he deserved to let his hair down with the boys. Most of his 'boys' weren't married, and most were younger than him.

Partying took his mind away from a reality he wasn't happy with, and sleeping with younger women who didn't require anything more from him than a good time was his way of distracting himself from deeper issues that had surfaced around the birth of his child.

I tried to focus on what was really happening, versus just getting stuck in his behaviour, which he was smart enough to know wasn't serving his life at all. Here was a man who had never been Fathered himself, and so, on a very deep level, he questioned if he had what it took to be a Father himself - especially when things got hard and real.

Here was a man who equated responsibility with obligation - and obligation, to him, made 'boring family life' feel like prison. Of course, when he wasn't showing up as he was needed his wife would rightfully 'get on his case', which reinforced to him that here was someone else telling him what to do, and demanding more from him than he felt able to give. He would react to this negatively and, in his mind, he would tell himself that she was the one stopping his freedom.

Really, he was avoiding being an adult at all costs. Grown-up commitments - paying a mortgage and having a child - suddenly overwhelmed him, to the point where he felt trapped. If you ever see an animal trapped, they will do whatever it takes to quickly escape - even if it's physically detrimental to them.

The constant partying and irresponsible sexual behaviour were like he had reverted from a 30-something man to an adolescent teenager. He left his wife to pick up the pieces of a young, shattered family while she was worked through her own heartbreak as the result of his betrayal.

I remember looking at him this particular day, and thinking the only prison he was in was one of his own mind, and the subconscious beliefs that were now destroying his life. I felt sad that his 'prison' went with him wherever he was, and that he didn't even realise it. It was absolutely nothing to do with his wife or child, but his own mind being a hostile environment – and the beliefs of deep unworthiness that had grown from his own, very unwanted existence. At the core of everything, he told himself constantly that he really wasn't good enough for the life he had always wanted.

An absent Father and an addicted Mother had once built the prison he resided in as a small child. Unfortunately, he didn't ever realise that for the entire time he had been an adult it was now only him standing inside the prison walls, and that he held the key that could open the door and bring him real freedom.

His ability to be something he never received, and the power to change the narrative of his story, were, in fact, in *his* hands.

This is something I've really pondered on when I hear of state services encouraging orphaned men (which is basically what they are, because they are parentless by absence or addiction) to do mandated parenting classes. I'm all for anyone learning and growing – especially in the area of parenting. Our kids deserve this. But I've personally wondered if the success rate would be higher if they taught these men how to re-parent *themselves* first. Because how can anyone really be expected to parent or nurture anyone else well, when *they* are emotional orphans themselves?

This is too often the cruel reality of the men I've met who feel trapped in a prison and unable to grow up. Their inner little boy is barricaded inside their hearts, stuck in the pain that first traumatised them, and now cannot grow up. That little boy really does feel trapped in a self-imposed prison of sorts, and I genuinely believe he wants so much to reach out beyond the prison bars to participate more wholeheartedly in life.

So, to those with an inner little boy stuck in a prison like I, too, was, I gently invite you to learn to speak with him, in the hope that you will now be able to give yourself what you did not receive.

This is a practice that I have done myself repeatedly for years now. Not only has it really helped me hear what my inner little boy is trying to say, but it's also helped him hear what he needed to hear a long time ago. The quicker you listen to him so he feels heard, the quicker he can leave his self-imposed prison, where he's been trapped for too long.

Once upon a time your inner little boy didn't feel heard, or seen, or loved, or wanted. And, over the years, you've built all kinds of prison walls around him to protect him from the pain of rejection, or disappointment, or the grief that your inner little boy felt when no one else around him protected him.

It was very clever of you at the time – you were doing your best to keep him safe. But now, as an adult, those walls you've carefully built to keep him safe only really keep *you* lonely and frustrated, unseen and unloved, stuck inside your prison. Walls like anger or denial you've built so high around him have kept your inner little boy trapped inside. He's even still the same age as he was when he was first hurt, because he's effectively been frozen in time, unable to learn anything new.

'If you are someone who sees your family life or relationship as a prison, then ask yourself why.'

And those walls now? They not only keep him stuck inside, they also keep out all the people you love who really want the opportunity to love you, too.

So whenever someone bumps into your walls and 'triggers' you, causing an overreaction from you (like when you yell or lash out), realise that it's only your inner little boy wanting to feel heard. He didn't feel heard then, and he's not heard now behind all of your walls. He's not really even angry – he's often just scared! So it's time now to sit with him and have a really good heart-to-heart conversation.

There are things he needs to understand, and how we can best help him to understand is to show up for him now and tell him something new so he can reclaim his voice.

It might go a little bit like this conversation I had with my own inner little boy:

> Little Scared Matt,
>
> You did your best, with everything you knew at the time; you did your best to survive. I'm proud of you for that. You didn't deserve what happened to you back then, and I'm sorry they hurt and humiliated you.
>
> Please try to understand that your parents had their own wounded little children within them. As a child you took everything they inflicted on you personally, as the truth about you, from the ones you believed should love you. You believed by the way they treated you that you were unlovable and unworthy.
>
> The truth is, Little Matt, it was never about you.
>
> You are so worthy and lovable. Your parents were just in so much pain that pain was all that came from them. And from this pain, your shame was created.
>
> But, Little Matt, you don't need to hold onto any beliefs that betray you or are no longer your friend. You don't need to be anything or anyone other than who you really are. You can wholeheartedly be the loving man that Little Matt always wanted and needed.
>
> This man is brave! He'll show up for you now, Little Matt, like no one else ever did.
>
> I see you. I hear you.
>
> I'm sorry it took me a while.
>
> You're safe now.

I love you.

I forgive you.

I thank you for your patience.

Matt

BROTHERS, IT'S TIME FOR our inner little boys to grow now. It's time for them to heal and live beyond their prison walls.

They're allowed to be seen by those who have shown you they love you.

You are allowed to be seen by those who have shown you they love you.

It's safe now to learn to let people in. If you can learn to apply boundaries instead of walls, you'll never have to live in a prison again.

Don't be scared to do this practice. Talking to the inner little boy trapped inside has been some of the most healing work I've done on my own journey. I'm not embarrassed, nor too proud to admit this, and in doing this work I'm doing the work of re-parenting myself. Re-parenting myself is me showing up **now**, and giving myself what I needed to grow that I didn't receive from my parents. It's me no longer waiting for or expecting any 'big person in my life' to give me what I can actually give myself.

Sometimes, especially while writing this book, I've closed my eyes and pictured myself as Little Matt. I can see my parents and my brothers, and watch all the interactions happening. I see my Mother in desperation trying to drink a bottle of bleach to end her life. I see my brothers kneeling on the ground with their arms in the air in front of our Christmas tree, staying like this for the duration of the game my Father watches on TV, because if they move out of this position, he beats them. I watch my Father kick our pet dog Rambo if he barks too much. I see how rough he is even with Great-grandma, how he forcibly grabs her arm and sits her down.

I watch and witness everything. I see the anger of the hostile environment. I see the pain and feel the fear. This was my childhood prison, so I give myself permission to feel what was. Sometimes I cry or feel sad. Sometimes I have a sick stomach seeing everything, but it's here that I accept what is. This is my story. This is where I came from. This is where I first learnt about life. Where I first felt fear. Where I learnt the feeling of humiliation, and learnt what shame physically does to your body. This is where I first learnt to hide at any cost, and to stay silent and shut down. This is where I cried under my bed alone. Here is where I first saw marriage, and where I learnt how abuse and love could co-exist together for years and years.

It's that co-existing that muddled many things for me. bell hooks puts it perfectly when she says in her book *All About Love*:

> ... abused children have been taught by parenting adults that love can coexist with abuse. [...] This faulty thinking often shapes our adult perceptions of love. So that just as we would cling to the notion that those who hurt us as children loved us, we try to rationalize being hurt by other adults by insisting that they love us.

IN ACKNOWLEDGING AND ACCEPTING all that I see, I take this vision of Little Matt. He's such a good little boy, but so scared. I tell him that I have come for him, and that I witness the tears that no one else ever saw. I tell him that things are different now. That I'm making better choices for his wellbeing and life. I tell him he never has to go back there, and that the home he lives in now can be the very home he always dreamt of. Where there's always nice food to eat; where it's safe and warm, with laughter and kindness. I tell him that – in this home – he's always protected and loved, and never humiliated. I tell him we have a whole new reality now.

I know there are moments when Little Matt will still get a bit overwhelmed. I know that even in this beautiful new reality he'll have moments of being afraid, where he'll want to crawl back under his bed and hide. He'll have moments where he wants to shut down and retreat – but I'll keep reminding him of his new truth. I'll keep showing up for Little Matt. I'll keep telling him who he is.

You are smart.

You are brave.

You are kind.

You are loved.

The very affirmations that I do every night with my own young children, I do now with Little Matt too.

I am smart.

I am brave.

I am kind.

I am loved.

I'VE LEARNT THAT by showing up for Little Matt practically, in simple little ways like this, I am giving him the encouraging, comforting, nurturing and affirming voice that I needed as I grew up. In this way I was starved and malnourished, so feeding myself these words is what I do now to re-parent Little Matt.

I've learnt other ways to show up for him now, too – things like having boundaries. When I grew up, I saw none. And I was shown – through moments where I was sexually abused – that people could, and would, take what they wanted from you with no thought to the way it damaged you.

Learning to say 'No' has been a big step for me in this journey of re-parenting Little Matt.

I know we've already looked at the difference between putting up a wall and setting a boundary with other people. But it's really important to understand and do, so it's worth looking at again here.

When you hide behind the wall, you are acting defensively: you are keeping people out so they can't discover who you really are. Essentially it is a negative, disempowering action. Whereas setting a boundary is something you proactively do. You survey the situation and then choose where people can meet you –

and you put in place consequences if they ignore this. If they step over that boundary – by disrespecting you, or ignoring your wishes – you can follow through with the consequence for this behaviour. This could mean you don't see them for a while, or you choose a way to deal with them that is safe for you. Boundaries put the power back in your hands, whereas walls just reinforce feelings of powerlessness.

It's things like understanding that I don't need to do all things for everyone, or that I don't have to agree to doing something like giving money just because someone in my family expects me to. It's a hard lesson for a Pacific Islander to grasp – trust me on that – and initially it was really hard because it seemed to be the opposite of everything I had been taught. But there's so much power in understanding my own sovereignty; the power and authority I have in my own life to make decisions that best serve my needs, and the needs of my children. My children directly benefit from my wellness.

When I fully understood the power of my own mind to re-determine what life I lived in, I became free to live where I wanted.

Was it my childhood prison where anyone could abuse me?

Or was it my new reality – the life I was creating now by the choices I made daily to show up for myself?

This revolutionised my experience of life.

I now live free.

Chapter eleven

She is not your lifeline

I WANT TO START THIS CHAPTER with a very real invitation to anyone reading this who is contemplating the idea of suicide. I've been there, and I know first-hand the state of mind you eventually get to once you develop a preoccupation with taking your life, of ending things once and for all.

I invite you to reach out to people in your community who can genuinely assist you with real solutions, so you don't have to struggle alone with the pain you are in. Keeping these feelings hidden only ever seems to magnify them, and causes them to fester away and grow bigger in the dark.

These feelings, which seem real and never-ending, need to be brought into the light for help to be able to reach you. The agony of rejection, disappointment or abandonment - the ache of uselessness, powerlessness, failure and self-hatred. All of these feelings seem so overwhelming, I know. You'd be surprised at how many men have shared these very feelings with me, thinking they are the only soul in the world who is struggling with the weight of the pain they are carrying.

You aren't alone, Brother.

And your past is honestly not a very good indicator of your future. My past is so vastly different from the life I live now, and it's not because I'm different or special. I was just proactive about finding the right tools and insights that I needed at the right time to address the pain I lived with daily.

Your future can be so different with some new insight and tools to cope with things in a healthier way. Healing and wholeness are available to all of us if we are prepared to do the work. No exceptions – because eventually we find what we seek.

But you do need to go to the right places for help and guidance, and *you* need to be the one doing the work, doing the healing.

Which is why I need to address you dumping this particular heavy burden onto your wife/partner/girlfriend, and treating her like she is the only lifeline available to you. This is simply not true or fair – and she cannot solely be that for you, no matter how hard she tries.

By all means tell her how you are feeling, but then also allow her (if she is in the position and mental state herself to assist you) to help practically, by finding qualified people, and other family members who can adequately support you. Having a village or a tribe of people to support you together is far more sustainable for everyone.

To illustrate this point I want to share with you a real text conversation that I had with the partner of a client of mine some years ago. She messaged me late one night in absolute desperation:

> **LILY:** Hi Matt. I'm so sorry to bother you, but I'm writing to you because I just don't know what else to do or who to contact. It's about Jake. I know he opens up to you a bit when he gets a cut, and he's not in a good place right now.
>
> **ME:** Hey Lily, I'm so sorry to hear that. What's going on, and where is he?
>
> **LILY:** I don't actually know TBH. I broke up with him last

night because I just can't take it anymore. I can't say or do anything to snap him out of his down buzz. Being with him is like being on an emotional roller-coaster. I can't do or say anything without setting him off worse. It's gotten to the point where I don't like leaving him, or even going to work. I'm afraid of coming home to find he's done something to himself. I now feel physically sick from the anxiety of it and I can't go on like this.

ME: Oh wow, that's so full-on for you. I'll call him and see where he is, aye? What do you think the heart of it is at the moment?

LILY: He's been depressed for a while now, as you know. I think it hit him hard when his Nan died last year. They were close and she looked after him for most of his teen years. But then it's just little things: he hasn't kept up his job – he started one which seemed good, and then said he doesn't like it, so now he stays at home playing games all day. He constantly accuses me of cheating on him or being interested in other guys. He checks my Instagram all the time. It's gotten so bad that I kept threatening to leave him, and every time I do he cries, says I'm all he has, and that he'll just take his life because he's worthless. I end up begging him not to and promising to stay with him. He makes me promise not to involve anyone else and says he doesn't want my family in his business, but I actually don't know what else to do. He says counselling is useless and he doesn't need it. He says he just needs me to love him and support him, but I don't know how to do that.

[A little while later:]

ME: He's not answering his phone. I've texted him to call me, though.

LILY: He won't. But he'll prob text me all night that he's sorry and he has to go, and please forgive him, blah, blah, blah.

ME: Do you feel he's serious? Has he ever attempted anything like that?

LILY: Hmmm – I don't know anymore. Part of me thinks he would do it one day just to prove he could. Like out of spite, after we fight he'd maybe just do it in the moment. But then another part of me wonders if this is just him manipulating me and making me feel sorry for him. He's never actually done anything, but he has been careless with too much drinking/taking party pills a few times.

ME: Do you want to be with him?

LILY: I feel bad not to! I feel bad to give up on him because we've been together for over seven years. I just don't know if I'm enough now, though, because he's not getting any better. If anything, the last year has been the worst. Actual shit. I had a miscarriage at the start of the year, 21 weeks along, and it was really hard for me, but he made it all about him.

ME: You can't stay with anyone because you feel bad, and you can't keep him alive either. At some point he's got to be open to receiving help. Is there anyone else he trusts or listens to?

LILY: Probably you. I know he respects you. He used to be close with my Mum too, but he's distanced her after we had this big fight after losing the baby. He just made everything about him. Mum hit him up and told him to pull his head in. Said that I needed him to support me, too. He then got weird with her, and told me he didn't want me talking at all to her about our stuff. It's really hard being stuck with just him and his depression because I'm so isolated.

ME: That sux. Sorry, Sis. I'm here if you need me to come over and see him. You aren't isolated. He has to realise that you do want to help him, but you can't do that alone. Sorry for your loss, too.

LILY: I do love him and I do want to help him to get help, but I just can't keep going how we are. Last night I finally ended things because he keeps texting me at work, asking me to come home early because he says he needs me. My boss is not so understanding – it's happened way too much. I don't want to lose my job, too. How would we even live? It's not like he earns any money. I got home and blew up at him. Told him not to text me any more at work. He said fine – next time he'll just end it. I'm so over the threats I ended up screaming and telling him to fuck off. Now I feel so shit. He left, and I haven't heard from him all today. I don't know where he would go because he has no friends!

ME: His phone is on, so that's a good sign. I'll keep trying to get him.

EVENTUALLY I DID GET hold of him. I went and met up with him for breakfast a few days later. He was embarrassed that she had told me, but he understood she was at the end of what she could manage.

I listened to him, and I heard a man who was really just a boy who felt unwanted. The only woman he felt had ever truly loved and nurtured him was his Grandmother, and she had now passed on. He felt that was her leaving him. The way he manipulated his partner now was really out of his own sense of inadequacy and fear that she would leave him, too.

All the suicidal threats came from a place of real hurt and an inability to communicate his pain properly, but he wasn't actually at the stage of attempting to take his life. He just wanted someone to take his pain seriously.

Jake's life also lacked purpose. He didn't have any goals, and he moved from job to job, uncommitted, as he had no sense of where he actually wanted to be in life. He felt jealous of his partner as she was doing a job she loved. He felt threatened by the fact that her life went on quite easily without him.

I asked him what he had wanted to be when he was younger,

and he immediately said 'a police officer'. I asked him why he hadn't pursued it, and he admitted that he had applied a few years earlier but had failed the literacy test to get in.

This setback had knocked his confidence hugely, and he felt stuck trying to work out what else he could or would want to do. Meanwhile, he would take jobs he hated and then not stick at them. Now the failure and disappointment he felt with himself had brought him to a place of unemployment, with no motivation for life, and depression, which was drastically affecting his relationship – the last good thing left in his life.

'She can't be the only thing you have to live for, Brother. We have to change that,' I said to him, and he agreed.

'Your past is honestly not a very good indicator of your future.'

From that point, Jake became committed to his own life. It was a slow journey, but one that I was so proud of. He started seeing a therapist, which he was resistant to at first. I asked him why he was so hesitant to seek help from someone trained to help with this specific problem. He said he thought counselling was only for crazy people, and he didn't want to sit around talking about stuff that made him feel sad and useless.

I explained to him that the grief he was feeling was a normal emotion, and, while it was allowed to be felt, it just needed some work processing and working through. I asked him whether, if he needed a major surgery, he would want to operate on himself.

He was puzzled and said 'No'.

I explained that we sometimes go through hard, emotional times where we really need professional help to work through it – just like if we physically needed help, and we would enlist the skills and expertise of a trained professional.

Brothers, it is not weak to seek help from trained professionals! So many of you suffer in silence, all because of something you have associated therapy with. Is it weakness? Some of the most successful men I know are men who have taken their mental health seriously, and have been brave enough to ask for help when they've needed to.

Just as many of us enlist the help of doctors for medical problems, personal trainers to meet fitness goals, accountants for our finances, there is nothing wrong with getting help from a qualified and experienced therapist who can assist you with your mental and emotional health. If you can't find the right person at first, keep going and try other people. You don't always take the first pair of shoes you try on, do you? That's because if the fit isn't right, you won't feel comfortable. You keep going until you find something that makes you feel comfortable and at ease.

There are also some people who get depression really badly, and it can slide into having suicidal thoughts, or feeling really exhausted and unable to cope with everyday life. This can be due to a chemical imbalance in the brain, and there's just no way you can talk yourself out of it. It's like having a constant hangover, and you can need professional help with this, too. There's no shame in taking medication for your mental health if you need to. I believe this is best done alongside other therapies, like talking, but nobody shames a diabetic for taking insulin to stay alive, and mental health medication is exactly the same. If this is you, it's time to get some balance back into your brain.

Along with therapy, Jake set some goals to do more things that made him happy. He decided to get back into his fitness, and started running daily, which he enjoyed. He also bravely set a goal to try to get into the police force again. He was so scared of failing this again, but I encouraged him to think of failure in a different way. Instead of telling himself that if he failed at his second attempt he was a loser, he would now tell himself that it was an opportunity to find out what he still needed to work on to pass. Passing the test or not passing the test, neither defined who he was as a person - it just indicated what job he could do. If he did fail again, then he would reassess, to see if it was still something he was committed to doing or if he would seek another path. Failure did not have to be fatal.

Sometimes we over-think things, or make them far more important than they are. We associate a particular job or opportunity with our worth as a person, and when we fail at that, we tell ourselves we are failures – which is not true. There will always be another job or opportunity. Some of my biggest disappointments have been with opportunities I really wanted but didn't receive. However, what did happen when I missed out was that I was available for something else, often even better! Instead of drowning in disappointment, I encourage you to learn to ask yourself: **What else does life have for me?**

The day arrived of the testing for Police College admission after a good year of solid work from Jake. He was in the best place he had ever been. Unfortunately, while he easily passed the physical, he failed the literacy test again. My heart sank when I read his text telling me he hadn't passed, and I worried about the effect this would have on him.

I met up with him a week later and, to my surprise, he was in relatively good spirits. He told me that after the news hit that he didn't get in, he thought hard about why he really wanted to be a police officer. It was mostly because he wanted to help young people like himself, who had been a bit lost. He then decided to start the journey of becoming a social worker, and enrolled in school to retrain. Within a few days of deciding this, an opportunity presented itself to him where he could work part-time in an after-school programme at a local gym with at-risk adolescent boys, incorporating fitness and life skills.

He was excited, and had happily given notice at his current labouring job.

Things were going really well with him and Lily, too, now that he had other passions to focus on outside of her. Along with seeking professional help, their relationship had gone from strength to strength, and they both remained committed to staying together. He realised that it was up to him to find more reasons to be alive than just her, and became engaged in his own life.

She couldn't be his only lifeline. That is an unreasonable demand of anyone. She was happy, however, to be part of a support system much bigger than just her, and for him to reach out and build a wider community. He realised this was the lifeline that connects us all.

I relate on a deep level, living here in New Zealand. As a Pacific Island Brother, I believe wholeheartedly in the Māori concept of *whanaungatanga*.

This very word has become the very essence of my business, and how I relate to all who are part of my barbershop community. This mighty word is all about being connected to each other. It's about building and maintaining relationships, where we work together to make decisions, and act in ways that support the betterment of the whānau (family).

But this can also be applied to more than just your immediate blood family – it can actually apply to your wider community.

How can we work together in collaboration to make decisions and act in ways that support a greater collective of people? What does this look like now, when most of us live in separate houses, with separate lives, and live very separately from each other?

'Shared pain is not only less traumatic, but it gives us reassurance that we are all in this journey together. If we find the courage to share, then we understand that we are far from alone.'

My parents were originally from the beautiful country of Sāmoa, and grew up in village life. My Mother was raised between two villages: Sapapali'i, on the north-east coast of the island of Savai'i, and Falelatai, a village west of Apia, the capital city, on the island of Upolu. My Father was from Nofoali'i, a village also on Upolu.

Most villages are where a wider community of people create their lives together, in support of and alongside each other.

They have their problems, too – no community of people is perfect – but did my parents ever feel the same isolation and disconnection in Sāmoa that they felt after moving to New Zealand? My Mother spoke of her time and life growing up in the Islands fondly, and spoke of her upbringing with her Father as a beautiful time where she was well looked after and cherished.

I've often wondered how life would have been for our aiga (family) if we had stayed in Sāmoa. Was Dad's alcoholism heightened by being in the unfamiliar land we ended up calling home? Would we have known in Sāmoa the same level of violence we experienced here? Would there have been a greater presence of community around us? Would this have made a difference to our life of violence, as we knew it?

Whenever I go and visit any of the Pacific Islands, I realise the life that my parents left behind. I understand their sacrifice and their desire to create a different life for us, but part of my soul longs for the community and connection that is part of our DNA, and part of life in the Islands. That's the essence I've carried into the DNA of my business.

I UNDERSTOOD THE DISCONNECTION felt by too many Brothers struggling alone. We were all seeking lifelines in one form or another – all with similar feelings of overwhelming depression and sadness.

It was late one night in the barbershop and I was completing my last haircut, on a young man named Liam. He seemed a little nervous at first, but by the end of the cut I felt we had connected, especially over our Fathers both loving their alcohol and how this played out in family life.

As I always do at the completion of a haircut, I showed him the back of his hair in the mirror with another, smaller mirror. I knew it looked good, and there's always that sense of pride you feel as a barber when you know you've given a blurry fade!

He lifted his head and stared into that mirror for the longest time, and then he started to cry. I asked him what was going on, and he told me that he had planned for this to be his very last cut as he wanted to take his life. He had planned to have it looking good for his funeral. But after our talk he had decided not to go ahead with it.

My heart dropped, and I grabbed him and hugged him tight while his body shook from crying so hard and he was trying his best to keep it in. I remember his words when he left: 'Thanks for seeing me tonight, Bro.'

I knew he wasn't talking about fitting him in for a cut.

That was when I realised that my barbershop wasn't just a place where people could come to have a good haircut or a chat. It was a place where men could come and start to heal.

SINCE I OPENED MY barbershop my mission has expanded. I've hosted and facilitated countless men's groups and hui (gatherings) all around New Zealand, inside prisons, barbershops and churches, and on marae. Similar to an Alcoholics Anonymous (AA) meeting, I usually start the group sharing part of my story, and then open up the space to hear many other stories of the men present. It always touches my soul when vulnerability is present, and people share what is true to them. Sometimes I witness the genuine surprise on a man's face after he shares something really hard for him, and then he sees those around him nodding in agreement, because they, too, have lived similar pain and struggle. Shared pain is not only less traumatic, but it gives us reassurance that we are all in this journey together. If we find the courage to share, then we understand that we are far from alone.

Suicide can never be reversed, and the pain is only transferred to those left behind trying to make sense of what is now too late to change. In the men's groups I have facilitated, I'm always reminded how much we need each other. The American civil rights activist and poet Maya Angelou once said:

> I don't believe an accident of birth makes people sisters or brothers. It makes them siblings, gives them mutuality of parentage. Sisterhood and brotherhood is a condition people have to work at.

Brotherhood is where we work to create lifelines between each other. In everything I do, *this* is the work of my life.

Will you join me?

Chapter twelve

She is not your hired help

IF THE ROLES WERE REVERSED, would you be happy to assume all the responsibility for her life?

With the March 2020 Covid-19 lockdown in New Zealand, when my barbershops were unable to open, I found myself at home full-time, appreciating even more the role of the stay-at-home parent. Sarah was studying full-time online for university, and co-ordinating our non-profit work projects, so I took over the tasks of entertaining and attempting to teach our children, along with cooking and cleaning the house.

The first four weeks were an eye-opener, juggling everything. I would often say to Sarah at the end of the day that I was exhausted by the sheer amount of energy it took to consistently occupy our children on demand. The word I would use to describe the workload was 'relentless'.

The relentless and never-ending tasks like washing (who knew we used so many items so often?) or making yet another meal (who knew that such small human beings could eat so much, so regularly?) meant that, by the end of my time at home,

I was looking forward to getting back to the barbershop because - truthfully - it seemed easier.

That's right. My job managing a heap of staff, running two barbershops, cutting the hair of all my clients, and listening to them share deep and personal things about themselves, along with teaching at the prison, seemed easier than staying home with my small children and caring for them.

That was when I think I truly grasped the magnitude of the role that, for generations, has been seen as 'secondary' or 'menial' or - to some - like 'a perpetual holiday'. In fact, it's an unpaid, full-time job, with no days off, where you are responsible for the wellbeing and survival of those in your care, but where this relationship is not reciprocated. Any relationship where you endlessly give with very little receiving will have a high potential for burnout.

I read in an article online that it was estimated that the job of a stay-at-home parent who took responsibility for the majority of the domestic duties was valued conservatively as a six-figure income. This was arrived at by breaking down the role into each task undertaken, and then valuing these tasks at what you would have to pay to outsource them. For example:

Cooking meals	→	hiring a chef
Cleaning	→	hiring a housekeeper or cleaner
Childcare	→	hiring a nanny or using a day-care service
Driving	→	hiring a chauffeur
Assisting children with homework	→	hiring a tutor
Doing laundry	→	using a laundromat or laundry service
Co-ordinating everyone's calendars	→	hiring a personal assistant

You can quickly see how that could add up if you had to pay a market rate for everything needed to organise a family and run a home. I definitely couldn't afford to pay my wife six figures – sorry, babe – *but* I can afford to be thankful and appreciative of the work she does every day, raising our children while I am at the barbershop, and for making our house a home. She is mutually appreciative of the work I do, and kindly offers me foot massages after I've spent a long day standing in the barbershop. (I would appreciate them more often, but take what I can!)

Mutual appreciation for what your partner brings to the relationship is something I think is essential to a happy life together. I can honestly say I have thanked my wife for every single meal she has ever cooked me. She says this is one of the reasons she loves cooking for me so much, and why she happily does what can often be a (literally) thankless task. Sarah puts thought and passion into the food she makes me, and, quite honestly, if all I have to do is say 'thank you' and tell her the meal is delicious, then the payoff is pretty massive for me!

When I think of coming home after a long day, I mostly arrive home to a clean, tidy house, happy children, and a home-cooked meal. Someone gifting me acts of service is the main way I feel loved, so having all of these things done for me contributes greatly to the love tank of my heart being filled up consistently.

Sometimes she jokes that if I had come home an hour earlier I would have arrived into chaos, so I appreciate Sarah making an effort to organise our home in such a way that it's calm and organised for me. I know that this is no easy task with the demands of three children and helping me with running our business. I appreciate that this isn't possible for other families – sometimes other things are a higher priority, like just making sure all the kids are fed and happy. A clean house isn't so high on the priority list. Everyone has a different set of priorities, and it's important to make sure your wife or partner doesn't feel like she has to carry this burden on her own.

As I mentioned earlier, growing up, I lived in a home where I saw my Mother do all of the domestic tasks. I didn't see any outward appreciation for anything she did from anyone; it was as if it was expected she should do all of this purely because she was born female. It didn't even matter when she worked long, tiring hours at the factory. It was her responsibility to come home, clean the house, and prepare all the meals. If these things weren't up to my Father's standard or liking, she would get a physical beating for it.

It makes me sad to think back and see my Mother live like this – she was basically nothing more than the unpaid help in her own home, with no appreciation shown for any of what she did for us. She was a slave to my Father's demands and desires.

'Our sons, and our daughters, deserve to grow up in a world where there are no stereotypical gender-based roles. This starts at home with us.'

I recall a time after my baby sister, Katherine, died at birth, and my Mother had come home from the hospital with no baby, but with all the physical effects from having just given birth. She was in our small bathroom, crying, bent over our bathtub filled up with water, washing our clothing as she always did. I watched her do this many times. On this day, it was spring and our house was cold. We didn't have a washing machine back then, and this was typically her task alone to have to do for us. I think this memory of this particular time is engraved in my mind because, even at that young age, I understood that there was no regard for her wellbeing. Even then I thought Dad was mean not to help her, especially seeing her physical discomfort. I remember Dad yelling at her, and cursing at her in the car on the way back home with no baby. All the while she sat there and cried. This memory makes me so sad now as a grown man.

I often wondered how her spirit survived this treatment.

At the time I was only four years old – my two older brothers would have been seven and nine. We had a younger brother who was only two who she also had to care for. There was no time for her to process her grief, and no one around to even care for her in this moment – just a steady stream of domestic chores requiring her attention and effort.

Sadly, this wasn't a unique situation in her generation. In a cultural sense, it was pretty normal, really: for that time and across multiple cultures all over the world, it was expected for women to do the lion's share, if not all, of the household jobs.

Fast-forward to now and we have more women working outside the home and pursuing their own studies and careers than ever before, but have we really changed the mindset we have towards each gender's responsibilities at home?

'If we truly value her, then we need to place a fair value on what she offers our relationship, home, and family.'

My job is to speak with men every day. I have a different client every 30–60 minutes. Many of my clients I have been cutting now for years – men from all walks of life and all ages – and it is so interesting to hear their varied thoughts and views of equality within their relationships, especially with regard to what he thinks her role as a wife and a Mother actually entails.

I had an interesting client once. He was in his early fifties, brought up in a white Afrikaans area in South Africa. He had lived in New Zealand for over a decade after relocating with his family for what he described here as a 'better, safer, life'.

One particular day while I was cutting his hair, he was complaining about a woman in the office where he worked. From what I gathered, she had a reception/admin-type role and he had a more senior position. He said they had exchanged words in the lunchroom because it had been left in a mess. He had told her to clean it up, and she had refused, saying it wasn't her mess to clean, and that she didn't even eat in there.

I asked him if he was her manager, or if she was answerable to him.

'No,' he said.

'Did you believe that it wasn't her mess?' I asked him.

'That's not the point!' he said. 'As one of the only women in the office, and being in such a menial position, she should take it upon herself to tidy things up when needed.'

'Surely everyone should be responsible for their own mess, though?' I asked him. 'Is it really fair that, just because she's a woman at a lower pay grade, she has to clean up after messy grown men in the lunchroom because they are too lazy to do it? I mean, if it's not in her contract, or part of her job description, why should she do it?'

At this point I sensed he was getting exasperated, and his white face was going pink.

He went on to tell me that women in New Zealand were too strong and argumentative for their own good. Apparently, they needed to know their roles, like the women he knew from back home! At this point I had to tell him that I, and many other New Zealand men I knew, really loved and respected strong women. Needless to say, the rest of the appointment was pretty silent and he never returned!

I don't mind conversations getting a bit heated - barbershops thrive with debate and banter - and I love to challenge viewpoints!

He brought up an interesting point to consider, though: what role is it that women *should* be fulfilling? And in the current cultural climate, where there are unprecedented advances for women nationally and internationally, are women really still seen to be responsible for tidying up after men who refuse to clean up after themselves? It was interesting discussing this with my wife when I got home that evening. She had a laugh at some of his comments, and joked that he wouldn't be equally matched to any woman she knew!

THERE'S A TERM THAT describes what it is when we expect the women in our lives to be on top of all of the 'stuff' of daily life, and that is *emotional labour*. It's not just having to do the work – she also has to try to manage everyone's feelings as well, including her own. I experienced taking on that role first-hand during our first Covid-19 lockdown, and, like I said, it is relentless.

Consider this:

- How do you add to your wife or partner's load of emotional labour?

- What do you take responsibility for that she doesn't need to think about?

- Are you both on the school's email list, so the school can contact either of you if anything happens with your kids?

- Do you both go to the school parent–teacher interviews, or do you leave 'that stuff' to her?

- Can you do a grocery shop and know that everything you pick out is what is wanted and needed that week?

THE ROLE I SEE for my wife is that of an equal. This is in every sense. I would be cutting in my barbershop for 40 hours a week, and in the early days of our business while I was at the barbershop she was the primary caregiver of our children when they were babies and being breastfed. We decided that our children wouldn't be cared for by any daycare or other outside provider for the first year of their life. This was a decision we made together with conversation around what I could offer.

Our eldest has just finished high school and is now at university, our middle child has just started primary school, and our baby girl is at daycare. While I'm working in the barbershops, or at a prison, Sarah is studying, or working at home on our businesses and non-profit ventures. She's also a part-time celebrant, along with assisting me in myriad ways with all the tasks I need to do for my work.

I might, in monetary terms, bring home the bulk of 'the food for the table', but it is Sarah who cooks the food and sets the table. Does earning the bulk of the family income entitle me to do what I want, whenever I want? The simple answer is 'No'. I couldn't do what I do if she didn't do what she does to keep us all running smoothly. Together, we form the partnership of what we desire family life to be for us.

Not everyone can afford to have someone at home, taking care of the children and running the household. In some households both parents work, in other households there's only one parent, so navigating the demands of everyone (adult and children) becomes harder. Working out what your priorities are to keep the household running is really important. Is it essential that you have a tidy house? Could you look at paying someone to clean it once a week, or once a fortnight? Who does the food shopping? Can it be ordered online and delivered at a time that suits? Who monitors what activities are going on for everyone, like sports or music or tutoring? Is there a family calendar in the house that everyone can write their activities on so that you are as involved and mindful about all the elements of family life as she is?

Based on the ages of our children, our situation is just what we currently do, and at some point in the future we will discuss what the new dynamics need to be, and we will change them to suit our mutual needs. It's important to us both that we meet the needs and desires of our children well, providing for them in ways that they deserve to be provided for. When the time comes, I'm happy to look at changing things up.

I have always seen Sarah's role at home as working for our family, just as I see my role in the barbershop as working for our family. I've understood that, outside of my hours in the shop, I'm a present and hands-on Father, just as she is a present and hands-on Mother. When I get home from work, we are both equally as responsible for meeting our children's needs and doing what needs to be done around the house.

For those Brothers who think their full-time job entitles them to a free pass around the house, I invite you to think again.

EVER SINCE OUR SON came along, I have said that I would be happy to be a stay-at-home Dad, because I truly believe there is no greater role than raising our children. My wife laughed, and said I would need to up my culinary skills before this can occur – but in my view you don't need to be a chef, or a fussy cleaner, to do this particular role.

A friend is a stay-at-home Dad to seven children. His wife has a very successful career, which sees her regularly travelling internationally because of it. My wife says he is a culinary food god who makes gourmet meals and homemade bread every night, the house is perfectly organised and looks like something out of a magazine, and the children are all well loved and cared for, with all of their various after-school activities orchestrated and co-ordinated by him.

This does sound amazing, and when she was first telling me about him I'll admit to thinking: 'I don't think I'm quite up to this calibre yet – I still spend three hours cleaning one bathroom, and any meal attempt I have made watching Jamie Oliver's video tutorials usually takes half the night and a trolley full of ingredients we'll probably never use again!'

But the response from those around him interested me most.

Sarah said it varies from sheer disbelief that this is even possible for a man to willingly want to do, let alone do so well – or there's an overkill on the flattery and praise that he gets (mostly from women) for doing such a task.

Yep, he gets over-the-top praise for the task of looking after his own house and raising and feeding his own kids. I mean, do women praise other women doing the same role quite so generously?

It was interesting to see what was reported in the media when Jacinda Ardern was elected as our prime minister, gave birth while in office and went back to work, while her partner Clarke assumed the primary caregiver role for their daughter, Neve. The comments ranged from sympathy for him having to do this (be a Father for his own child) to apparent outrage that she was not taking care of her own child, and could she really manage having such a role (as prime minister) while also being a Mother?

Sarah was beyond frustrated with that dialogue, and wrote this Facebook post on 19 January 2018:

> Reading the out-dated opinions of silly ignorant people in comments on our Prime Minister's baby news truly shows the state of what women in 2018 actually have to deal with.
>
> It's absolutely bloody pathetic.
>
> 1. Yes, she is Prime Minister – elected for three years to serve our country.
>
> 2. That doesn't mean we own her body – just like our respective workplaces don't own our bodies when we sign up to work for them.
>
> 3. That doesn't mean we get a say in her decision to have a child with her partner. Planned or unplanned, it's really not our business.
>
> 4. She has already stated that her partner will be a full-time stay-at-home parent to their child. Why can't we celebrate a Father choosing that incredible role versus trying to make the Mother feel it should solely be hers?
>
> 5. Why is it inconceivable that she can run the country and be a Mother to her child, when our last PM was a Father to 6 children, and the one before that was a Father to 2 children. I never heard anyone question their abilities to do both.
>
> 6. This is 2018, and most of us are juggling parenting and work–life balance. That's just reality – because gone are the days where the majority of us can afford to live on one wage!

7. Women are *capable and qualified* to be boss leaders and kick-ass Mamas! That's just how we roll!

Seriously! Her body! Her choice! Give the poor woman a *break* with the judgement and let her get on with it!

#WahineToa #WelcomeTo2018 #YouGotThisJacinda

OVER 300 PEOPLE 'LIKED' her post. It reflected the frustration felt by many that clearly we, as a society, weren't as evolved as we thought we should be.

As Sarah pointed out, Jacinda had only an hour to decide to become the leader of the Labour Party mid-election. She then had just over a month to campaign, and to completely turn around the election, which she did. Her beloved Grandmother died only three days before the election. She then discovered she was pregnant during the coalition discussions; her cat was run over and died on her first day back in Parliament. She carried on pregnant, as a new prime minister, giving birth to her daughter while in office, and took only six weeks off before resuming her role as prime minister again full-time.

Jacinda proved many times over that she could do the role more than competently, yet the media commentary that was on repeat was always asking how, still, she could be a more effective working Mother.

WHILE ENORMOUS STRIDES ARE being made in the advancement of women everywhere, I wonder if we, as a society, have made the same advancements in our thinking on the place and role of women in our homes. If we truly value her, then we need to place a fair value on what she offers our relationship, home and family.

She is far more than merely 'hired help' to tick off items on a chores list that I would rather not do. She does them all, repeatedly, out of a genuine love for us. My wife is my co-pilot, my partner-in-crime, and the person who co-creates everything our home and family is. This role is of such high significance to the overall wellbeing of everyone in our home, and yet is still viewed somewhat dismissively by some arrogant men who make comments like 'What does she do all day?' or 'She's lucky she gets to stay home all day while I'm working hard to provide for our family'.

The truth is, if you are a Brother who has grown up with this kind of belief about women and their 'place' at home, think back to where and who you learnt it from. Were these the comments your own Father made? If so, it's now time to update your ideas and change the narrative so we (and our attitudes) can evolve. Our sons, and our daughters, deserve to grow up in a world where there are no stereotypical gender-based roles. This starts at home with us.

Sarah once asked me if I saw her as my equal, and I thought about what that looked like in real-time in our relationship. I think we both bring different elements with the same magnitude of importance and value to our partnership. We are both very strong-minded, opinionated and passionate, but also open to learning, getting it wrong and re-learning. It makes for a relationship that I feel transcends the traditional archaic framework society has too frequently painted of what a marriage should look, feel or sound like.

Since I married Sarah, I've questioned extensively that corrupted patriarchal mindset that still exists in so many arenas of the world, and I've concluded that the only reason any male would have for not wanting an equal in his partner is because of a deep-rooted fear that, somehow, he is not enough. Once we truly comprehend we are enough just as we are, we have no need to ever dominate or control anyone else.

In fact, it's the complete opposite – we *yearn* for our equal.

Chapter thirteen

She is not your punching bag

NEW ZEALAND HAS SOME of the worst domestic violence statistics in the world. Call it what you will - domestic violence, intimate partner violence or family harm - it's a devastating reality. One in three women have experienced physical and/or sexual intimate partner violence in their lifetime. That statistic goes up to 55% if you factor in emotional or psychological abuse. One in two Māori women have experienced intimate partner violence, and for Pasifika women and Pākehā women that drops to one in three. One in ten Asian women report the intimate partner violence they have experienced - but we don't have any idea how many assaults go unreported. One in seven young people report being harmed on purpose by an adult at home. Half of all homicides are family violence, and half of all intimate partner violence deaths happen when a couple separates.

Studies have also found that experiencing or witnessing abuse or domestic violence in childhood increases the risk of becoming either a victim or a perpetrator of intimate partner violence as adults. We have set ourselves up for intergenerational violence to carry on unless we do something about it in our lifetimes.

Some of you won't understand, but some of you reading this will know exactly how it feels to witness for the first time the terrifying moment when you have no power to protect your own Mother from your own Father. The helplessness and fear that merge into one sick, horrifying feeling of dread will never be forgotten. It's the moment when you know there is nothing safe about your world, and there really isn't anywhere to go or to hide to avoid it. This is your life, and all you can do is somehow, by whatever means possible, endure it.

ONE OF THE EARLIEST memories I have, one that I will never forget, is from when I was only about three years old. My Mother was standing in the kitchen, and in utter desperation, following another heated and furious argument she'd had with my Father, she screamed that she was going to kill herself.

She grabbed what was closest to her at the time, which happened to be a bottle of bleach, and she tried choking herself with it by savagely pouring it down her throat quickly, in an attempt to drown herself.

I didn't comprehend fully what she was doing at the time, but I remember standing there so still, absolutely petrified, seeing this all unfold in front of me with no idea of how to stop it. I was crying and begging Dad to help her, while in front of me there she was, with bleach pouring everywhere. It was at that point I recall him storming into the kitchen and hitting her savagely across the head. She fell on the floor, and he grabbed bottles of water from the fridge and started pouring them into her mouth while forcibly holding her down in an attempt to make her choke and drown.

My two older brothers came running into the room, and tried to get my Father off her. But he was too strong, and they were only children themselves, not even in double digits. Eventually he left her laying there, a pitiful heap on the floor, and my brothers lay alongside her, crying. Then she saw me standing a little way away, stuck and crying, unsure of what I should do, and she beckoned for me to come over to her. I did, and all three of us boys lay on the floor, clinging to her, crying.

The fear of that moment has never left me, and today I think of the Little Matt then and want to hold him close – as I do with all the 'Little Matts' everywhere now whose homes are battlegrounds and who have no safe place to go. I want to warn him that things in his life will get so much worse before they ever get better, but to hold on. That eventually he will have the family life he wanted so badly.

To any man inflicting this kind of abuse on those he says he loves, I want to ask you this: **What emotion are you avoiding feeling *so much* that you would rather terrify your children, and terrorise the woman you say you love, than face up and feel it?**

For my Father, his rage was a culmination of many things; grief in losing his Mother at a young age, but also great disappointment at how his life had turned out. I don't believe he ever really let go of the life he hoped for but never lived. To this day, I don't even think I genuinely know my Father for who he is. He's this complete enigma of a man, whose alcoholism and rage, along with poor mental health, utterly submerged his personality.

Mix all this with his daily alcohol addiction and you have a man who easily lashed out whenever he was triggered. And the triggers were numerous. Anything imaginable could trigger him to resort to violence. If my Mother or us kids didn't perform or behave in a certain way, the food not being cooked to his liking, the house not being clean, something at work happening that left him feeling inadequate – any of these things could trigger him to explode all of the pent-up frustrations on us, his family. We were his punching bag. It was as if, to him, violence was the only acceptable way he ever could ever express his feelings. I'm sure he wasn't the only one who felt that way in our wider community.

Our childhood was absolutely riddled with his violence. My first Christmas memory is my Father picking up the Christmas tree, drunk as he always was, and beating my Mother with it.

My older brothers, again, tried to protect her by lying on top of her, to somehow take the edge off the beating.

One particular day my Mother dared to try to escape him, and walked to the bus stop directly outside our house. As soon as she got there my Father stormed out of the house, punching her in the face in broad daylight, with no regard whatsoever for any neighbours seeing it. She fell to the ground, and he dragged her by her hair along the ground back into our house.

People saw, but did nothing. I saw them watching out of their windows, too scared to get involved. I've seen Mum being run over by Dad in the driveway, and chased around the house with a machete. I've seen her blood on the floors and smeared on the walls. I've seen him stomp on her head while holding her down.

My Mother had countless black eyes - often both eyes at the same time. Off she would go to church with them, and to get the groceries, and even to drop us off at school. Still, no one in our world said or did a thing. It was like people saw the prison we were living in, but they just stood there staring, unsure who they should tell about what they were seeing. Such people can also become part of the overall problem by refusing to say anything to those involved, or to the right authorities, who may have stopped any violence continuing.

ANGER IS SUCH A misunderstood emotion, especially with us males. There are times when anger can be used positively and can fuel us to make positive changes, but it's actually what is commonly referred to as a *secondary emotion*, because it's often fuelled by other emotions. Anger can be a mask for our pain. And underneath this mask we have a whole host of other emotions and feelings masquerading themselves as anger:

Fear	Not being heard	Humiliation
Frustration	Inadequacy	Grief
Disappointment	Rejection	Sadness
Abandonment	Shame	Trauma

HALF OF THE TIME, with the men I'm speaking with, I don't actually think they are really angry. Their anger is just a secondary emotion which is easier to deal with than what is causing it. If they actually chose to sit with their anger long enough - instead of simply reacting to it - they would see that their anger or rage is a diversion from the real cause, their *real* emotions - their disappointment, fear or grief. Situations or circumstances around them are in fact triggering these *primary emotions*, which they just don't want to feel. So they shut them down - as painful as that is - and summon up that guard dog named 'Anger' to protect themselves from feeling.

Instead of taking up the invitation to feel our emotions for what they are - an indicator that something is wrong and an opportunity to grow beyond our pain - we find it easier to blow up and lash out. But while it *seems* easier, it really isn't. In the long term the denied emotions all build up into a seething hot volcano inside of you, just waiting for the next thing to trigger you into blowing off a little bit of the steam.

So to the guys who think they 'feel better' after they have hit someone, or blown up, you probably do with a bit of a cathartic release - but it's only temporary. It's a bit like the geysers in Rotorua. Every so often they have a good blow-out, and then gradually some more dirt or mud gets piled up on top, and the pressure starts building until they blow again. That's you and your anger. Make no mistake: there is *always* a next time, so you are only ever prolonging the inevitable.

I've chosen now, in my thirties, the son of an angry alcoholic, to come to that place of feeling, and travel down a different path from the path continually shown to me throughout my childhood. I do this for myself, so that I can live the life I always wanted, but I also do this for my wife and our children, so they can live the life they deserve. My family are my greatest motivation. **Stop and think about what's going on in your life. What would motivate you to change?**

While I have never once physically assaulted my wife in any kind of way, I know for damn sure that my words have been used as daggers aimed at her heart. They are especially potent to my wife's spirit, because *words of affirmation* are Sarah's primary love language. They are how she is nourished and uplifted, so when words are used to do the opposite, I see what they do to her and it feels as if I've physically wounded her.

When I see the hurt I've caused, I've had to grow my capacity to humble myself and apologise to her. I'm proud of the progress I've made in this area, perhaps because it has been so hard to rewire. I'm faster to apologise than I was at the beginning of our relationship, and I regularly 'bend my knee' to her.

She is not my punching bag, and she should also not be a dartboard where I fire derogatory words at her heart with a triumphant 'bullseye!' Actually, over the time we have been together, she has become the greatest and wisest confidante I have ever had. So instead of lashing out our frustrations on our partner, why can't we learn to share them with her? Instead of reacting to her, why don't we remind ourselves that she stands there, waiting to be let in, when everyone else has long since gone? Why are we so afraid to allow vulnerability to be a part of how we respond in our relationships?

I shared a poem on social media, to challenge this thinking:

> Brothers, why do you refuse to shed a tear?
> But instead break your fists
> on anything that gets in your way?
> You prefer broken bones,
> than to expose your broken soul?
> You'd rather your heart
> haemorrhage through your hands
> instead of your eyes?
> It's time for a new way, Brother,
> Let your tears flow free
> We must *feel* to *heal*.

WE HAVE SO MANY other emotions inside of us, other than just anger. So why has anger been the only acceptable one to express for men? If we really think about it, no other basic human emotion has caused so much pain and suffering all over the world like anger has. Think of the wars fought, the refuges everywhere housing women and children bruised and battered, the accidents caused by road rage.

I've met a lot of angry men. I've lived with angry men. I've worked with angry men. I cut the hair of angry men. I know angry men. I've been abused by angry men. I've been, at times, an angry man.

I will admit that sometimes the easiest, most natural response is to flare up and get angry. I can think of a very specific example where it could have gone one of two ways.

Anyone who owns a business - especially a barbershop - knows that having staff is probably one of the hardest things to deal with. I've had staff steal from me, cause scenes with their ex in the shop, not show up to work on our busiest day with clients booked in back-to-back, or show up drunk or high. I've had staff be blatantly disrespectful, or just ignore any boundaries or rules I might enforce. I've even had a grown-ass man basically have a temper tantrum in the shop in front of clients because I told him 'No', leading to him quitting on the spot, and then going around slandering me, my family and my business to anyone who would listen, including clients.

Honestly, I've had it all, and through it I've learnt to see through a lot of bullshit that insecure boys - who have never had the skills to grow up and behave properly - dish out. So I genuinely feel real empathy for women who are in relationships with these men, and have also had to grow a thick skin in the process. My word of advice for anyone attempting to start or run their own business is to truly learn not to take things so personally. It's usually never about you, and 99% of the time it is about issues the person has in their life that need addressing.

SOME TIME AGO I had a staff member take the cake in disrespect. He had been with me for years and I had invested a lot into him. By that, I mean I had gone above and beyond to give him opportunities beyond barbering in the shop, which he also got paid well for. He enjoyed free trips away regularly, including going overseas to learn new skills. I did this all in the hope that he would learn to invest in himself once he saw that someone had invested in him.

I saw a lot of potential in a boy who on the outside seemed like a mess. I saw how he was raised, and I wanted to give him the opportunity that I wished someone had given me. I had built up my business in a garden shed in a poor neighbourhood, starting from the ground up, and overcoming the many obstacles and struggles one inevitably encounters in business. I had a deep desire within me to make the path easier for other younger barbers coming up through the ranks, and to give them the opportunities I never had. I regularly remind myself that I'm in the business of people, and that it is *people* not *profit* that I am investing in daily.

Unfortunately, investing in people means you don't always receive a tangible return that you can see straight away, and in this particular case, I made a mistake.

He came up to me one day, when the shop was full and I was cutting my client's hair, and waved a single sheet of typed paper at me before walking away. He was resigning, without notice, to go and work for another barber. For me, the worst thing was that it was clear he definitely hadn't written the note himself, and that, after everything, he wasn't even respectful enough to sit down and have a face-to-face conversation!

I was in shock. Only a week before he'd told me during a training session that he was in it for the long haul. I felt genuine disappointment that he hadn't kept his word, and that my efforts on his behalf were unappreciated. He didn't finish out the week, and on his way out he took some of my clippers with him. Then he was pictured on the social media of another barbershop that same day, smiling and wearing their uniform.

Sarah had warned me earlier that he could not be trusted, as had other family members. I had not heeded their warnings, and genuinely saw him as a little Brother who just needed some love and support to be what I believed he could be.

I must admit that, more than any other staff member leaving

over the years, his leaving was a definite blow to my heart, and it took a few days for me to pick myself up from this loss.

Initially, I felt so *angry* with him. I felt I'd wasted so much time, energy and love on this man. Then I thought about it, and I realised what I really felt was hurt, sadness, disappointment, foolishness – and betrayal. My pride had taken a hit. I had taken the word of a man, invested in him, and he had taken me for a ride. It was also a harsh reminder to me of people in my past doing similar things to me, and mistaking my kindness for weakness.

'Is anyone actually ever loyal to me?' I wondered.

'What emotion are you avoiding feeling *so much* that you would rather terrify your children, and terrorise the woman you say you love, than just face up and feel it?'

I knew that how I would go forward from this was up to me, and I played out all the various scenarios in my head. Would I enlist the help of my more 'gangsta' clients and pissed-off Brothers who were angry at his disrespect too, to teach him a lesson with a fist in his face?

Would I stop future staff from getting close to me, like he was?

Would I take out my frustrations on those closest to me – like my wife – who had so annoyingly foreseen this happening?

All of these responses were right there, ready to go, and it was on one particular day, at the end of the longest week, when I hit an all-time low, and I got into an argument with my wife. I couldn't tell you what kicked it off, or even what we argued about, but I remember snapping at her rudely and raising my voice. I stormed off outside to unload the car, and then came in and was crashing about the kitchen loudly so she would know how I felt. I went over to the corner of the kitchen – angry – ready to pounce on whatever she dared say to me. A stubborn flush of anger and frustration had come over me, and I was in no mood at all for a calm discussion.

My back was to her, when I heard her walk in, and I braced myself for battle. Suddenly her hand was on my back, gently rubbing me. Then I heard her say: 'I'm sorry he hurt you like that, my love. He has no loyalty to you because he has no loyalty to himself.' The walls of anger came tumbling down faster than I had erected them. I turned and faced her, put my head on her shoulder and sobbed like a baby!

Oh, the tears. Tears that to some could be seen as shameful or weak were simply tears that needed shedding to release the emotions I was rightfully feeling. Would it have been manlier if I'd punched the wall, or continued to yell out my frustrations and hurt at her? I don't think so. Why is it that we believe violence is more acceptable than tears? Tears are far less damaging to you and everyone around you!

For those of you who don't know, tears - and crying - are scientifically proven to be good for you. Emotional tears release and flush out stress hormones from your body. It's a self-soothing process that calms the nervous system, and helps your body to rest and digest. Crying dulls the pain you might be feeling by releasing oxytocin and endorphins - these are the 'feel-good' hormones that calm you and give you a sense of wellbeing. It seems crazy, but crying can instantly improve your mood, because you literally feel a sense of relief - like a dam has burst. Crying can help you process and recover from grief. It restores emotional balance in your body, and it can also be a sign to others that you need help.

Of course, if you find that you're crying more often than normal, or you find it hard to stop, you could be heading into depression, in which case it's best to seek help from a doctor or therapist. This also applies if you're thinking about death or suicide. Ignoring these feelings won't help in the long term, Brother, so please reach out.

The tears had to come, and come they did for me that day, standing in the kitchen, crying on my wife's shoulder while she gently rubbed my back, and told me the truth of the situation.

That image of her rubbing my back is immortalised for me. It's a visual reminder of her compassion and humility that is forever engrained in my mind. Remembering it helps me to catch myself in moments, too, where my anger has begun to get the best of me, and I start to react instead of respond. I think about this moment, and the ways she could have reacted to me. Sarah could have met me with the same negative energy I gave her. But she didn't. Her response became an invitation for vulnerability, and a chance for me to heal.

TOO MANY ANGRY MEN believe anger is the *only* acceptable emotion for them to feel, and sadly go through life expressing their anger in forms like violence or verbal abuse.

But here's what I've learnt.

I've found that when we have the **courage to sit with our anger**, and actually find a bit more about it, we can find out what is driving it. For me, when I've sat with mine, I've learnt that anger surfaces when I don't want to feel the *real* feeling inside - which is often something I have felt at other times in my childhood or past. I'll give anything not to have to feel that way again. So when my closest relationship with Sarah triggers in me feelings of:

  not being heard
  feeling inadequate
  feeling stupid
  feeling exposed or humiliated
  feeling betrayed

it's all too easy for me to immediately react in anger.

I learnt, growing up in my home, that it's more than okay for a man to be angry. It's okay and acceptable to lash out, because the feelings I feel need some kind of release, right? But the reality is the feelings aren't really released, or processed, or healed. The real feelings hide away while my **angry mask** takes over. I encourage any Brother who brings out his angry mask in such moments to do what *any* human being should rightfully be able to do. Cry.

I cried all over my wife's shoulder that day.

Sometimes the tears can last a while. But I find them to be far more cathartic than yelling or snapping at the people I love.

Men cry. Women cry. Human beings cry.

It's a natural bodily function of ours.

Let's have the courage to cry if we need to, my Brother. I don't know who first came up with the idea that we should be frightened of our tears, but it's time to let our tears flow. Sometimes, just like in childbirth, the waters have to break so we can experience new life.

ANGER IS A NORMAL emotion that can help us – if we learn how to manage and channel it well. It is important to learn how to express anger in ways that are appropriate for you, while keeping yourself and others around you safe.

If you have ever felt so angry that you can't control yourself, this is a sign that you have a problem managing your anger. Other signs include:

- getting irritable and overreacting at the smallest things

- anger being your first and often only 'go-to' response

- getting aggressive, violent or nasty when you get angry – yelling at others, or insulting them (this is verbal abuse, and it's not okay either)

- needing alcohol or drugs to calm or relax yourself.

ANGER CAN ALSO BE a sign that you're dealing with a lot of stress and things are feeling unmanageable inside. Observe how your body reacts to others and to various situations. If you feel your energy is always heightened and aggressive, then it's time to look deeper and ask yourself if you can identify your anger and notice what is triggering it. While you do this inner work, it is wise to consider putting strategies in place so you are not a slave to your anger. These include:

- Breathing deeply. Using breathwork techniques is one of the simplest ways to regulate our emotions. It's a technique I discovered through a good friend of mine named Lino, with some of the work he does with his men's movement in Australia. We have access and the ability to do this anywhere.

- Learning to take yourself out of any situation in which you feel out of control with anger. You cannot expect to police others' behaviour, but if you feel triggered to the point of aggressively lashing out at others, then it's time to know you must leave the room or situation.

- Learning how to talk to yourself when you're angry. Talk to the boy within yourself. What has frustrated or disappointed you? Be kind to yourself with your words. Too many of us behave like angry children having tantrums because we haven't learnt any better ways of coping.

- Finding ways to manage your stress in consistent, regular ways before angry outbursts occur; techniques like breathwork, exercise or meditation can really help to stabilise our moods and emotions so we aren't living in constant highs and lows.

- Seeking professional help if your anger is getting out of control. There are all kinds of support groups available online or in person. I believe we always find what we seek. It's possible for our rage to not be the master of our life.

Chapter fourteen

She is not yours to control

AS A BOY who grew up in a world that was so out of control with violence and abuse, I know, without doubt, that it instilled in me a permanent sense of uncertainty that made me question whether my very basic human needs, including safety, would ever be consistently met. I felt powerless in the unstable environment that I was forced to grow up in. This has had lasting repercussions that can still affect me now - as a man in my thirties - seeking to subconsciously control my environment as an adult.

We keep doing what we think we need to do to survive, until we learn that the survival mechanisms we once used are no longer helpful to us or to the life that we want.

If you are not aware of the attachment theories described by leading developmental psychologist John Bowlby, I invite you to research his theory on attachment. It says that young children need to develop a secure bond with at least one primary caregiver for optimal emotional development to occur. If there are attachment issues in childhood, this can often lead to difficulty forming healthy relationships as adults. Children generally thrive when their caregiver can competently and consistently meet their needs, and so many of us who were abused instead of nurtured by our caregivers go on to have emotional problems in adulthood.

As adults, we can often be unaware of how our childhood experiences can influence the relationship issues we currently have. And in my own quest for understanding and answers for why I would react the way I do in certain situations, I had to go right back and learn where things started for me.

Now, I feel I need to make a disclaimer here.

Going back to and understanding our childhood stories might feel like we are disrespecting our parents because of the emotions that can arise in making sense of everything. In some cultures there is a taboo or an unspoken rule 'not to go there'. Growing up in a traditional Sāmoan home, we were taught to honour our parents above all. Unfortunately, honour can masquerade as having to pretend things didn't happen that did, or not speaking about the things that happened when they really need talking about.

But until we acknowledge these stories, how can we change them?

Sometimes, when we go back to make sense of our stories, we can feel angry or really sad about what occurred, and it can be too easy to blame our parents for their shortcomings which we perceive have ruined our lives.

In my journey I've come to understand with my own story of origin *not* to blame or shame my parents, but rather to understand, make sense of it, and heal so that these behaviours don't get passed on to my own children.

It's through this lens that I have come to view and try to understand the hugely problematic issue of *coercive control*.

What is coercive control? It's a form of abuse that uses a range of different behaviour patterns to instil fear and compliance in a partner. Men (and it's usually men) try to control their wife or partner by limiting access to money, monitoring her communications, isolating her from her support network, name-calling or putting her down, reinforcing traditional gender roles, gaslighting (making her question her own sense of reality), making jealous accusations, trying to turn her children against her, and controlling aspects of her health and body. People under this type of control are scared to put a foot wrong, question everything, and become timid and fearful.

There are many men who would believe that this book or any of my work is not for them. They would say that they don't need it. Brothers in my own extended family whose harmful behaviour has been witnessed by many would say this. There are men who would never see themselves as abusers or perpetrators of violence because 'I've never hit her!'

I've worked with men who describe their harmful behaviour as 'relationship issues' – alluding to what is happening as something they both should take accountability for. But when I hear what is occurring in that relationship, I know, without doubt, that it is he who must acknowledge his abuse of her.

So let me be clear with you all: **You can be abusive and never hit her. You can be abusive and never physically leave a mark.**

ABUSE IS FAR MORE than just physical violence; it can also be attempting to control another grown adult by manipulating them, making them feel scared or guilty, or by blackmailing them into doing what you want. None of this is acceptable, it is abusive and creates an unequal power dynamic in a relationship. In some parts of the world, like England and Wales, these forms of abuse are illegal, but in other parts of the world such behaviour is condoned and even built into legislation. Women and children become chattels of the husband and Father. They have no say in their lives at all.

Is this what you want your relationship to be?

If you are not in a reciprocal relationship of mutual trust and respect, where both partners feel they are freely able to leave without threat to their safety and wellbeing, then it is not a relationship. One of you is a prisoner and the other is their jailer.

Now, I can understand why someone who has come from a situation like my own childhood can become controlling and become that jailer.

But while it's understandable, Brother, it is also completely unacceptable.

When you have felt powerless in your life, you can easily fall into the trap of wanting to feel powerful - and when we crave power at any cost, then **someone else must pay that cost**.

By holding so tightly onto power, we think it will somehow bring control to our chaotic world, and we won't be in a position where we can be hurt again. But the reality is that we have become controlling, and we are now compromising the freedom, safety and wellbeing of another.

We have now become that abuser.

We have become who we don't want to be hurt by.

We have become the person we were once scared of.

You think you feel more powerful, but it's a delusion and it exists at her cost. She doesn't feel powerful because - in your attempt to control her - you have taken over her autonomy and taken away her right to choose.

Love without choice is not love. Such relationships are not an equal power balance. Relationships that are healthy mean *both* parties are healthy and empowered.

Both have equal authority.

Both have a voice.

Both are confident.

Both can have strength.

Both can have vulnerability.

Both are heard.

Both can make decisions.

WHEN WE RUN AROUND trying in vain to control our world and the people in it, to alleviate the chance of anyone controlling us or hurting us again, we are, in fact, running on a hamster wheel where we get nowhere.

It is impossible to fully control the world around us.

It is impossible to fully control anyone else.

It is impossible to ever be completely in control of our lives.

In my barbershop I facilitated a therapy session with a group of men, and we discussed the concept of *power over* versus *power with*. We agreed that power in itself is neither 'bad' nor 'good', but rather it's how we decide to use and distribute that power that matters.

When we have a relationship that has a balance of power, and we actually share power between us, this empowers our partners and ourselves to be our best selves and live our best lives.

We agreed that this was the best-case scenario, because when we don't share power, and one member of the relationship is controlling or coercive, we buy into the concept of 'lack' and we start to believe that there is a limit to how much power we can hold onto. In this instance we believe there will never be enough power, and attempts to control our partner or wife can become more coercive and controlling as the relationship progresses.

Here's an example to illustrate how a *power over* relationship starts, continues, and may eventually end. No one wins. Please think about *what is happening for each of them* as you consider their stories.

Jack grew up in a dysfunctional home where his critical Father ruled with an iron fist. He regularly bullied his family with angry, verbally abusive outbursts, which terrified Jack's Mother. She struggled with depression, as well as having to care for Jack and his two younger siblings. As much as Jack tried to protect his Mother and younger siblings, Jack's Father would regularly beat them all, and things would end up worse for Jack if his Father thought he was being disobedient or disrespectful.

As Jack grew up, he resented how his Father treated him and made him feel, and Jack eventually in turn became a bully to his peers. He liked how he could feel powerful in this space, and find some sense of control, which he never felt at home. Many of Jack's peers found it easier to be friends with him and do what he wanted rather than risk being bullied by him, too.

Jack continued to put himself in situations where he could feel powerful and in control. In the workplace this was rewarded, and eventually he found himself in lucrative senior roles where he was responsible for many staff. Again, his staff found it easier to do what he wanted rather than risk being victimised or bullied by him, and he developed a reputation for unfairly firing staff he didn't like.

Through work, Jack met Hanna, and he decided that he loved her enough to marry her. Hanna was sweet, but had her own history of childhood sadness. When she was only nine her Mother had left her Father - and her. Because she was scared of being abandoned again, Hanna found it very difficult to say 'No' to people, and became a 'people-pleaser' - never having strong opinions and always putting other people first. This trait worked well in her relationship with Jack, because, as long as he got what he wanted, things seemed to go really well between them. There were many positive attributes about him, too - he was charismatic, confident, charming and financially successful.

It wasn't too long before they married, but even then Jack insisted on eloping even though Hanna told him it was important to her to have her Father and sister there. One day Jack 'surprised' her with a date to the registry office, where he told her he just couldn't wait another day. Hanna was surprised that all the paperwork had been done even after she had told him how she felt. But she was surprised and a little delighted that he'd gone to such efforts to marry her. She figured this was *true love* and it was normal to feel so overwhelmed.

Once they were married, Jack declared that he wanted to have two children immediately, and encouraged Hanna to leave her job as soon as she became pregnant. He told her he was happy to provide for her, and look after her and their children. He took control over everything, including their finances, while Hanna focused on raising their children. Jack professed to Hanna that she was 'his world', and life went smoothly as long as Hanna gave him what he wanted, when he wanted it. Throughout their relationship Jack never bothered to ask Hanna what she wanted, and she was scared to voice any opinion, in case he got angry or upset.

However, after years of having her emotional needs discounted, Hanna began to look for things to fulfil herself. She wanted to be able to see her friends and family without Jack getting angry, and she wanted to start working again, now that the children were at school. So she found a job at her children's school that enabled her to only work during school hours and term time. She was delighted, but Jack was angry and resentful. He saw this as belittling him and his ability as a provider. He said to anyone who would listen: 'Why isn't she grateful to me for the life we have? I give her everything she needs.'

'In my journey I've come to understand with my own story of origin not to blame or shame my parents, but rather to understand, make sense of it, and heal so that these behaviours don't get passed on to my own children.'

As a result, Jack gave Hanna the silent treatment for two weeks after she accepted the job, and picked a fight with her on the morning of her first day. This made Hanna feel sick and anxious, but she really wanted the opportunity to work and do something for herself. Then Jack began to make impossible demands, and their heated arguments became more frequent. He complained about her cleaning and her cooking, and said she didn't make the same effort for him or their family since she'd started work. He kept control over her money, because it was paid into a joint account that only he had the password to, and so she had to ask him every time she needed money.

One night things escalated and he threw a plate across the room, smashing it, and frightening their children. Hanna threatened to leave the house and take the children to stay somewhere else for the night. Jack pushed her up against the kitchen wall, put his face right up to hers and hissed: 'I will never allow *you* - who is such a *bad mother* - to take *my* children anywhere!' The children witnessed all of this.

Later on, when the heat had gone out of the situation, Jack

cried and apologised to Hanna for his behaviour. 'I just want our kids to have the kind of family life they deserve,' he said.

Knowing his childhood story, Hanna felt sorry for him. She vowed to try harder and make more of an effort to keep him happy – even if she wasn't happy herself. She made up his favourite meals, and planned activities she knew he would enjoy doing on the weekend, so that he could see and, she hoped, appreciate the effort she was making with family life. Putting her own feelings aside, she even had sex with Jack whenever he wanted, even though most of the time she didn't feel like it. Even so, Hanna felt more and more resentful because, despite all her efforts, Jack continued to pick fights over nothing, and would never say anything positive to her or about her. And she never knew when his next fight would come.

One day Hanna was stuck at work and asked a friend to pick up the children and take them home. By the time she got home, Jack was there and he was furious. He grabbed her by the arm and marched her to the car, pointing to her petrol gauge. He screamed at her: 'Where the fuck have you been? I know how much petrol it takes to get to school and back! Who have you been with?'

Then he started to track her cellphone. 'I won't be made a fool of!'

Jack began to manipulate their children, telling them that their Mother didn't care about them now that she'd started working again. Hanna overheard her son say that he wished his Mummy didn't work, and Hanna started feeling guilty for doing something she enjoyed, because it seemed like she was abandoning her children, just like her Mother had abandoned her.

In order to keep Jack and their children happy, Hanna decided to quit her job, but it didn't take long for her resentment to bubble up, as she realised that her whole life revolved around keeping Jack happy, and that her feelings or desires didn't matter to him at all.

When Jack was made redundant from his job, they all suffered. He found it difficult to get a similar position and salary, and took on a role which paid almost 25% less. Jack became even more temperamental and short-fused with Hanna and the children. When Hanna offered to go back to work, Jack blew up, screaming: 'You constantly undermine me and my abilities, and I am sick of it!'

Jack blamed Hanna for everything: he said she made life harder, and all the daily arguments were her fault. Everyone felt miserable, including their two children who witnessed his daily outbursts. Because Jack had taken a pay-cut, he became even more controlling around their finances. Hanna had to justify every item on the grocery bill, and had to ask for permission to take the children to the doctor. He even made her justify how much petrol she needed in the car to take the children to school.

Out of desperation, Hanna reached out to her sister and finally told her what had been happening. Her sister was supportive and told her that she had been quite worried about her relationship for some time. 'He doesn't hit me, and I should really try to make things better at home – it's partly my fault,' Hanna said. Her sister offered to help her and the children move out for a bit, until something permanent could be sorted. Hanna wanted to leave, but was terrified about Jack's reaction and how that could affect her sister.

The next day, as Hanna tried to take the children on an outing, Jack and Hanna had another heated argument. It was the last straw for Hanna, and she told him she wanted to separate.

'If you leave you will have nothing to live on! You will have *no* money, and no judge will give you custody of those children because you're such a mentally unstable woman! Why don't you just fuck off and leave me with the kids? You're just as bad as your Mother!'

By this time Hanna was completely emotionally and physically exhausted, and felt that she didn't have the energy or the means to fight Jack in court.

After this incident, Jack monitored every move Hanna made, and threatened to keep their children from seeing Hanna's sister because she was a 'bad influence' on them, trying to break up their family. In an attempt to protect her sister, Hanna decided to distance herself from her extended family, but this only reinforced

Hanna's feeling that she was alone, and her mental health suffered even more.

In her worst moments, Hanna contemplated suicide, not because she wanted to die, but just because she couldn't see a feasible way out of what felt like an endless hell. She regularly planned how she would kill herself, in detail. Most days she felt spaced-out and was barely functioning in her own life. This increased Jack's verbal abuse, and Hanna felt unable to be fully present for her children. Meanwhile, the children had begun to exhibit noticeable learning and behavioural problems at school.

This was the *hell* of coercive control that Hanna and Jack lived, along with their two young children.

Ask yourself: is this the life Jack really wanted?

Is this life really what anyone wants?

A suicidal wife?

Children whose happiness is so severely compromised that they can't learn properly at school?

A marriage where your wife can barely function?

A life where you must force those in your world to stay?

My Brothers, forced love is not love. It may be all kinds of things, but it is not love. And I write this genuinely from a place of understanding. When you have grown up with little or no control over your basic safety and security, then I understand the allure of a *power over* relationship. I can understand why it's appealing to attempt to create as much control in your life as possible. And it may temporarily compensate for feeling helpless.

But this is not what you really want.

What you really want is to be really comfortable in your skin, even when you have no control. When you can understand and *make friends* with the fact that, in life, we can only ever control our own reactions and responses. There is real freedom in accepting this.

If you think about it, in most circumstances what happens – including the actions of other people – is out of our control. Even the most organised plans can change without notice. If we are to survive and thrive in this world, we must understand the notion of *adaptability*. When we learn to be flexible to the ever-changing landscape of life, we realise the power in being able to move and bend, as we need to, for we are not immovable mountains.

She is not yours to control because she must belong to herself. She must belong to herself in her ways, and you must also belong to yourself as an independent, conscious entity who deserves your own sovereignty.

Belonging to ourselves is when we are free to decide *how* we live.

You are worthy of a woman who is free enough to choose you with her whole heart, and co-design a life together with you.

Learning to master our reactions so that they become responses is really what we need to control. Controlling our reactions comes down to deciding *who* is in charge.

Ask yourself:

- Is my ego in charge?

- Is my pride the boss of my life?

- Do I always need to be right?

- Do I always need to be in charge?

If the answer to those questions is 'yes', ask yourself one more question:

- Am I open to this changing?

IF YOU RECOGNISE THAT you are replicating some of those coercive control behaviours, please talk to someone about getting help. Recognising those behaviours in yourself is the first step on the pathway of growth and real change.

I gently encourage you, in the moments of chaos and frustration, and those times when you feel out of control in life, to align yourself with what is true and lasting. When I feel this way, I ask myself these questions:

- Is this more important than what my children will believe about me if they witness this?

- Is this something that will matter at the end of my life?

- Is this how I want to be known or remembered by my wife/partner who signed up to live life *with me*, not *for me?*

IN EVERY SINGLE MOMENT when I have pondered on these questions, I am reminded that nothing matters more to me than my children's experience of me. And when I remember this, I remember who I am, and I see clearly my place in this world as their Father, their role model, their teacher, and their safe place.

When I live in alignment with *this* calling, I find I have no need to control anything.

So, my Brothers, are you open to surrendering the need to control everything?

And, are you open to surrendering the overwhelming desire to control her?

Chapter fifteen

She is not your doormat

A KEY COMPONENT of any healthy, balanced union is that it's *reciprocal*, meaning that there is give and take, and that both people in the relationship get their needs met. A partnership - with *both* voices being heard and valued - doesn't work if she is just an object for you to metaphorically 'wipe your feet on'.

Let's start with her ability to say 'No' to you. 'No' is a perfectly acceptable answer in a reciprocal, functional relationship, but in many dysfunctional relationships, serious conflict arises if she dares to utter this small but mighty word. For example:

No, I don't want to have sex with you tonight.
No, I'm not able to cook you a meal right now.
No, I don't feel comfortable with that.
No, I already have plans.
No, we can't afford that.
No, I'm not cleaning up after you.
No, I don't want to do that.
No, I don't want you to sleep around on me.
No.

ALL OF THESE ARE perfectly acceptable responses. Brother, if you really want – or expect – a doormat for a partner, then I challenge you to search within and ask yourself why.

- Are you threatened by a woman who can stand up for herself?

- Do you feel insecure or abandoned when a woman tells you 'No'?

- Are you intimidated by a woman who has her own life, plans, opinions, thoughts and feelings, and who doesn't allow herself to be controlled or manipulated by you?

LET'S GO DEEPER. WHEN she stands up to you, or says 'No', what is the *real* feeling you are experiencing at the heart of it? And when was the first time you remember feeling that way?

For many men I converse with, they don't initially have the emotional vocabulary to even go there. Many men are so used to shutting off these feelings, they can't identify at all what's going on within themselves. It's a permanent state of being totally unaware. It didn't feel nice or good when someone told him 'No' or 'Not right now' in the past, so now he goes through his life refusing to allow this to ever occur in his relationships, by having a tantrum when she does say these dreaded few words.

I always start with breaking it down with him like this:

- Do you think that her saying 'No' to you really deserved such a strong emotional outburst from you?

- Did her saying 'No' to you really warrant the abuse or violence that you reacted with?

- Let's address the real feeling underneath your reaction to her saying 'No': does her saying 'No' bring up feelings of rejection or abandonment?

- Does her standing up to you challenge your ego or even your masculinity?

IN ALL MY EXPERIENCE with men, there are the same key fears or unbearable feelings at the core of every one of these tantrums that need addressing and working through. Remember: what we don't transform, we inevitably transmit. To transform things that are so unbearable to us that we will do anything within our power *not* to feel them - including controlling or manipulating the woman we say we love - we must first identify these feelings and be aware of what triggers them.

To assume that we can go through life controlling everyone around us just so we don't have to feel what really hurts is craziness - and it's exhausting.

I have an example of this exact behaviour in my own family. In this relationship he has all the control of their finances. His partner literally has to ask for money each week to be transferred to her to pay for basics, like groceries. He has all the control and makes all the decisions.

One day she decided to stand up to him, and calmly (and very thoughtfully) explained why there needed to be a more equal approach to ownership of their finances. She pointed out that they had been together for over a decade in a partnership. They both worked to bring income in for their family. They both valued raising their children in the same kind of way, and she had never done anything that warranted him removing her as a partner or equal in their financial affairs. She clearly asked for a joint account, where she had access to their joint funds, and didn't need to ask his permission to access their money for things like groceries. She said she felt it was fair to still discuss bigger purchases, but paying for things like groceries or the doctor's bill, she felt she shouldn't need permission.

I thought that sounded very fair and very clear.

He did not.

He had a meltdown.

The verbal abuse started. 'You dumb bitch! Why the fuck

would you think you could even do this? You can't even organise the house let alone balance the accounts!' (Yes, these were his actual words!)

The manipulation started. 'You're so fucking ungrateful! You think I want to do this? I'm doing you a fucking favour here. You've got it so damn good. I'm over here slaving my ass off making sure we are in the clear here!'

His undermining her and her capabilities started. 'You wouldn't know the first place to start! You're not the smartest fucking cookie, are you?'

He attempted to tow her back into line so he could control all of their finances, and therefore their relationship, keeping her right where he felt she belonged.

On the doorstep.
Never questioning his authority.
Never asking for anything he didn't want to give.
Never sharing her opinion or her reasons.
She was his doormat.
And he wiped his feet there often.

I ASKED HER IF she'd had enough yet. She asked me what I meant.

I said: 'At what point is this all too much for you to live with? How much do you have to sacrifice of yourself in order to allow him the control of your relationship?'

She thought hard. 'I guess I love him, and at the beginning - because I had never had another relationship - I just thought this was what you did. I didn't mind so much then. I thought he was just very traditional, and liked to provide for me and take care of all the details. He is a good man. He doesn't ever hit me or anything. Now, ten years on, it just feels like I'm trapped. And I really hate having to ask him for money to buy the basics!'

'Are you willing to bring this subject up again, knowing full well the kind of reaction you are probably going to get from him, but this time actually enforce your request with a consequence?' I asked.

She swallowed. 'Ah . . . like what?' she asked.

'Well, he's clearly not open to negotiating your relationship with a conversation where you tell him explicitly that you aren't happy with how things currently are. He has a tantrum, he abuses you, and you shut down and allow his behaviour to continue – even though it upsets you. It seems to me like you feel undermined, not valued, and you know your partnership isn't equal. He doesn't hit you with his hands, but his words hit you. That emotional blackmail takes its toll. Are you prepared to enforce what is rightfully yours now, and possibly leave this relationship if he refuses to give you financial equality?'

She looked at me for the longest time, then uttered the word her partner hated her saying the most.

'No.'

'I have seen so many things over the years that women allow from their partners, because they are so convinced that if they love them enough their man will eventually change. It is truly astounding. Men like this don't change until they understand the consequences of their actions.'

She said 'No' to me, and 'Yes' to staying in a marriage where she still doesn't – to this day – have any financial say whatsoever. She stayed because she came from a home where she witnessed her parents staying together through 'good times and bad'. When you come from this, you sometimes feel obligation or duty to stay, even when things are more bad than good.

Her husband, of course, had his reasons for controlling her the way he did. There are *always* subconscious reasons that can justify all of our conscious behaviour in our own minds, but until we check our subconscious reasons, our unchecked beliefs will rule our lives – and not always in the best way.

I asked him once why he controlled their finances so tightly, after I had observed some particularly bad behaviour of his towards her at a family function. His response was matter-of-fact. He didn't see there was a problem at all with him controlling her this way, because he just didn't trust anyone in this area of his life.

'Why?' I asked.

'My Mother was a gambler, and as children we had to starve while she went off and did what she did. I'd be stupid to trust a woman ever again with my money.'

'But your wife isn't your Mother, and you are robbing her of the chance to be your equal partner in life by living like this. You are robbing yourself. She's so scared to upset you that she says nothing, but lives with resentment toward you. Is this what you really want? A doormat that is too scared to call you out on your behaviour?' I asked.

He shrugged and stayed silent. He had suffered no consequences from her regarding the way he treated her, so what was his incentive to change? He got everything he thought he wanted. He was in control.

I have seen so many things over the years that women allow from their partners, because they are so convinced that if they love them enough their man will eventually change. It is truly astounding. Men like this don't change until they understand the consequences of their actions.

If he gets everything he wants from her, while she lies dormant at that front door of her own life as his doormat, why would anything ever change?

CHANGE IS WHAT HAPPENED to a man I knew well when his wife left him. For their entire marriage, he had cheated on her and lived his life selfishly, with little regard whatsoever for her or their children. She finally decided to leave him, after years of family members and friends encouraging her to do so, when she discovered while pregnant with their third child that he had given her chlamydia, something he had unknowingly picked up when being unfaithful to her. She was devastated to discover this halfway through her pregnancy, as their newborn baby risked also becoming infected during delivery and developing other health problems. This meant that she finally saw the impact his actions had not just on her, but on their children, too.

It was the final straw, and at 30 weeks pregnant she packed up her stuff and moved in with her parents. This took huge humility on her part, as they had never liked or approved of him, and she felt embarrassed that it had taken her so long to leave.

Initially, she understandably felt hurt, broken and rejected. She wondered if she had done the right thing for their sons, as he seemingly didn't care, and went about his life as if her leaving with their children didn't affect him. 'Would he even show up for the kids now?' she wondered, and felt guilty that leaving him meant that her children wouldn't have a Father at all.

She had their new son and tried valiantly to rebuild what she felt was a completely broken life. It took some time, and I remember feeling for her as she quietly went about rebuilding her life, finding a job, getting into her exercise and finding her feet. About a year later, I remember seeing her at a community event and thought she looked really good - happy, and like something had changed for her internally.

I got talking to her and asked how she was going. She said she was content with where she was at, and that the kids were thriving; she had found a job she enjoyed, and things were actually going well with her parents. She had also really gotten into going to the gym, and used it as stress relief and a way to feel strong. Ironically, she said that once things had stabilised for her, things had gone downhill for him. He suddenly had an epiphany about what he had lost, so he started trying to win her back.

She had told him in no uncertain terms that a real apology actually looked like changed behaviour - not just for her, she stipulated, but firstly for their children. He had to step up for them and for himself. She said she was tired of being a doormat, and she wouldn't allow herself to be this now in their co-parenting relationship. In fact, this wasn't going to be tolerated in any area of her life, and he had to step up or step away. He chose to step away in the end, and, unfortunately for them, saw less and less of their children.

THAT'S THE THING ABOUT a doormat. It stays there outside at the front door of its own life, weathering all kind of storms that eventually take their toll. A doormat always has multiple people walking all over them, because the way they show up in their relationship is generally how they show up everywhere else. In a sense, a doormat has resigned themselves to this being their particular role in life.

There are many reasons why a woman becomes a doormat. Sometimes it's because she's had an abusive upbringing, and being a doormat is a safe and familiar place. Sometimes it's because she's scared of losing what she has. If he holds the keys to all the money, has the house and the cars in his name, and he works full-time while she's at home or works part-time, she will feel trapped. How can she afford to go out on her own? It may have been a long time since she experienced independence, and it is scary for her. The thought of trying to leave him is overwhelming, so she stays in a place where she knows she can exist – as the doormat.

A doormat needs someone to walk all over her, and if that someone is you, you have to step back and pay her some respect.

So, my Brother, here's my challenge to you.

- Why can't you be challenged?

- Why don't you think you deserve an equal partnership with a woman who can, and will, challenge and grow you?

- Why do you desire obedience and submission instead of loyalty and genuine respect?

Because you don't have genuine love if she's forced into a life of permanent obligation to you. It's not honour if she has no other choice but to comply. It's not pleasurable for her if she doesn't consent. It's not a partnership if she has no voice. It's not healthy if she can't say 'No'.

You need to understand that what you are in is not a relationship. If she wants to leave you, but feels too scared to for whatever reason, then you, my Brother, are her jailer, and your home is a prison.

To be with another soul is really an honour. It's a privilege to share space and be allowed to journey together. Every day I wake up and marvel that my wife chooses me. Every day I feel grateful that she chooses our life together. There are a hundred other places in the world that she could be, yet here she is, choosing to share herself with me. Allowing me to share myself with her. Choosing to cherish me, honour me, be loyal to me, and respect me.

It wouldn't be the same if Sarah was forced into any element of our life. It wouldn't be the same if I emotionally manipulated her into staying, or if I physically beat her into never leaving. It wouldn't be the same if I controlled her in every possible way until she was little more than some robotic servant. If I did these things, I would never know whether she was really here with me out of love – *or out of fear*. I would never experience the freedom that holding our relationship with open hands brings.

There is a relationship analogy that talks about holding sand in our hands. If held loosely, the sand stays where it is – but the second you close your hand and squeeze tight to hold on, the sand trickles through your fingers. You might retain some of it, but unfortunately you'll lose most of it.

How many of you are stuck in relationships where you have held onto your partner so tightly that she can barely breathe? And how can she be who she was meant to be if she can't breathe? Is this really what you want for your life – and for hers?

Why are you denying yourself a chance at an equal partnership, where you share the load, and share the rewards of a fulfilling relationship?

It's not easy to examine yourself and change the way you operate. If you've been doing this for a while, you will probably both need professional help to illuminate the blind spots. There are things you can both unlearn, and steps you can take to rewire your brains. It will take time, and a lot of effort. But it's worth it. Imagine the amazing life you could share – together.

Sarah chooses me in the good times, and also in the times when life is far from easy. I feel a sense of overwhelming gratitude that, through all the seasons of our relationship, and in the dark depths of my own inner work and healing, I've learnt, and truly understand, that for it to be considered actual love, one must be free to choose.

She's free to leave, so I'm honoured she stays.

If love is a choice, then ask yourself honestly: Is she *really* free to choose you?

If you were given the choice, would you choose you?

And finally: **Do you really choose yourself?**

Chapter sixteen

She is not your competition

Chapter sixteen

She is not your competition

HAVE YOU EVER BEEN around a person who has to beat you in everything? No matter what you do, they have to somehow 'one-up' you. If you are running a five-km race, they are running a ten-km race. If you are talking about a recent vacation to Hawaii, they casually mention they were there *three* times last year alone. If you've lost weight, they've lost double the amount!

While it's exhausting to listen to, it must be even more exhausting to be that person who feels they have to out-do every other person they are around. I imagine that to have to come up with all the ways you can possibly be better than everyone else must be pretty time-consuming.

Bring that into your relationship, and instead of believing she is on your team, and you are progressing together in life as partners, suddenly she is your competition or – even worse – your enemy! I know of relationships where, out of his insecurity, she is not allowed to earn a higher salary than him even though common sense says this would benefit them both.

That seems so crazy, right? Surely you'd be happy that more

income is coming into your home? It benefits your family as a whole. But imagine being a woman who isn't *allowed* to progress through her career, as she should be able to, for fear of 'showing him up' or highlighting his inadequacies. It seems crazy, but it occurs in relationships all over the world.

Right now I'm thinking of a guy I know whose wife has turned down three promotions for a job she is exceptionally good at. Not only that, but a few years ago she had an opportunity to do her Master's degree, fully paid for by the company she worked for, because they wanted to further invest into her. But because of him, she turned it down.

He had told her in no uncertain terms: 'You don't need to waste your time doing shit for an extra bit of paper that you don't even need!' He deemed any pursuit of this nature 'selfish' when she had other responsibilities – to him and their child.

Her disappointment was very real, but she put on a brave face and told us all that she couldn't fit it in anyway. I've known him since high school, and this guy has always had an inferiority complex. He was super-competitive at school, but never quite good enough. He never made the top-grade rugby team. He was average in every subject. He was never 'cool enough' to hang out with the 'cool guys'. As an adult in his thirties he was onto his third career – and he'd never done exceptionally well in any of them.

It got to the point where he actively put down more-successful people around him in a bid to feel better than them. I genuinely felt for him. I understand what it's like to want to be good at something, and most guys I know do take a certain amount of pride in their work. To have such little success for your efforts when you try so hard would be discouraging for many of us. Society puts a huge pressure on people to work all the hours they can and to be successful, and men have the stereotype of needing to be 'a good provider' shoved at them, which can be hard if your wife or partner earns more than you do.

One evening we were all at a birthday dinner together when a mutual acquaintance innocently triggered a conversation that I knew wouldn't end well. She worked for the same company as his wife, but at a different branch, and excitedly said to her: 'Congratulations! I'm so inspired by your example!'

He immediately looked up from his meal and said sharply: 'Congratulations for what?'

I could see his wife looking at her friend wide-eyed and nervous, silently begging her to not to say anything more.

Oblivious, her friend went on: 'Did she not tell you? She's up for a company award! Her stats are some of the best in the country. It was shared on a staff email last Friday!'

He shook his head. 'Nah, she didn't say, but I've been so busy with work myself that we've barely seen each other this last week.' He laughed and proceeded to talk about his job.

I couldn't take my eyes off his wife's face. It was as if she was trying to make herself smaller and smaller so she didn't diminish *him* - the guy who needed every inch of attention the room could provide him, in a desperate attempt to validate himself. It was painful to watch, and I decided I needed to follow up with a private conversation with him.

A month later an opportunity came when he asked me if he could book in for an early-morning haircut before he had to head out of town to a family wedding. I was booked out, but offered to come into the shop earlier than we usually open on the day he was flying out, to give him a cut and shave. He agreed and I met him there, thinking to myself that this was the perfect chance to talk to him alone, since no one else would be in the shop.

I had my blade on his neck when I brought up his wife's nomination for the award, and because of the position he was in, he couldn't move. He opened his eyes and looked up at me.

'Bro, do you realise how you come across whenever your wife is being recognised for her hard work? It kinda comes across like you are jealous of her success,' I said.

I stopped blading him so he could respond.

'Jealous?' Then he let out a little snort. 'Bro, I'm not jealous at all. She does her thing, and I do mine!'

'Yeah, but that's not how it comes across, Bro. It seems like you aren't happy with her succeeding, and my bet is that's because you aren't succeeding how you wish you were,' I said, as I went about cleaning up my tools.

'I am, though,' he quickly replied. 'I'm doing real well, and I don't care what she does. If it keeps her happy, then all good.'

By now he was sitting up straighter in his chair, and he clearly wanted to dismiss this conversation.

I shook my head.

'Bro, honestly - you should hear yourself. It's so obvious to people all around you that your wife is really good at what she does and, somehow, you are threatened by that. Why do you refuse to encourage her, or even be happy for her? I don't know who you need to prove what to, but I can tell you that cutting her down isn't proving anything, other than that you are insecure.'

'Bro, honestly - I came for a haircut, not a lecture. Just make me look good for this damn wedding!' He said this jokingly as he closed his eyes, and leaned back in the chair in an attempt to halt any further conversation.

I got back to work and finished him up. I knew the conversation wasn't going anywhere, and he wasn't ready to hear the truth. Part of my job as a barber is to listen, and listen some more, and only say something when the time is right. I've learnt that timing with men is everything. And I've learnt to trust life - in as much that people know enough about their bullshit, and when they have had enough. If you go on at someone before they are ready and willing to hear what you have to say, then it's just noise. We had a relationship that was pretty straight-up, so I was comfortable in leaving it for a bit. I knew it wasn't the end.

About six months after that appointment, his wife asked Sarah to meet for lunch at a café. Almost immediately after they sat at a table she said: 'I think I'm going to leave him.'

'Why now?' Sarah asked.

She said she just couldn't continue on the way things were going.

'I love him, but honestly, I'm sick of not being what I could be. I got offered another position, and I really want to take it! I thought about just not telling him, but then I'm living with a man and he doesn't even really know me - or my job. I don't want to be dishonest with him, but I also don't want the constant battle. Anyway, I did tell him, and he instantly got annoyed at me, saying it was his turn to get ahead, and that we can't both be career-focused, because who is going to focus on our daughter? And even then, I'm like: but when has my work ever made her suffer?'

Nothing he said to her made any sense, and all his excuses did was further highlight his insatiable need to be better than her. For her, the worst part had been when their daughter heard their arguments, and when she had time alone with her Mother had asked her: 'Why doesn't Daddy like it that you are smart?'

When Sarah recounted their conversation, I decided to try once more to have another conversation with this guy. If he wasn't careful he was going to lose his family – all for the sake of his ego. I went around to his house when I knew just he would be there. He had avoided going on holiday with his wife and daughter, saying he had to work. By now he hadn't seen them for almost two weeks. He had also avoided me since the last haircut, and had been getting cut by other barbers in the barbershop, telling me he couldn't get in with me since I was too booked up.

He was sitting on his back deck with his feet up, drinking a beer, when I arrived.

'Living the life, aye Bro?' I said.

'Yeah, something like that,' he responded, and offered me a beer.

'How's things been, anyway?' I asked, as I sat next to him.

'Alright,' he said, but I sensed from his tone that the truth was far from that.

'Missing the girls yet?' I said, sipping my drink.

He let out a heavy breath.

'Everything's fucked!' He banged his beer down on the table. I sat there quietly waiting for him to go on, and after a long moment he did.

'I miss my girl. And I do miss my wife. This is the last thing I wanted. I know I have my issues, but it's not really that bad – is it?' He stared at me with a look of defeat in his eyes.

I got the message. It was time to get real with my Bro.

'I think you have to honestly ask yourself if you'd want to stay with someone who not only didn't encourage you to be the best version of yourself, but who also tore you down whenever they felt shit about themselves. Is that a relationship you'd want to be in? Is that a relationship that is going to get the best out of you? Your wife has covered your ass for long enough now, and it's come to the point where she's done! Do you honestly blame her?' I said.

'No,' he said quietly. 'I'm just tired of being a fucking failure. Nothing I do is ever good enough; it doesn't matter what it is. Everything she does she's good at - she has no idea how it feels to be someone who fucking tries so hard but still gets fucking nowhere! I don't blame her for leaving. She may as well leave me - everyone else has!'

And there it was.

'Bro. Is this about your Dad? Are you still waiting for him to come back and give you his approval?' I asked.

'Him? *Him?*' In spite of his vehement and bitter tone, he started to tear up, and began wiping at his face furiously.

'I just wanted him to say *one time* that he was proud of me, but do you think he ever did? From the time he left us, I wanted to make him proud of me so he would come home. But I wasn't fucking good enough for that, so he can fuck right off and *get fucked* with his fucking stupid new family!'

By this stage he was full-blown crying and simultaneously yelling. I reached over to him and pulled him in for a hug. Now he was wailing into my neck, his whole body convulsing with his sobs. I held him tightly for a long time until he calmed down.

'Bro, you're going to have to let go of needing his approval. He's never going to give it to you. Your worth as a person, and your value as a man, can't be in his hands a moment longer or it's going to destroy you. The thing is: you keep missing the point, and getting everything wrong.'

He blinked. 'What do you mean?'

'Bro, your wife is not your competition. In fact, no one else is your competition. Not your friends, not the guys at work. None of them! You are only in competition with yourself, and who you were yesterday. All you have to beat is that. If you learn something every day, then you are better than you were yesterday. If you act in a more loving, kinder way towards your wife, then you are better than you were yesterday. It must be exhausting for you to be running a race with people who just aren't your competition.'

'Not my competition? What do you mean by that?' He looked genuinely puzzled.

'We're all on the same team. Lots of people forget this as they go about life. You're on the same team as your wife – in the fact that you both want to raise your daughter to be the best she can be. It makes no sense to compete with someone who is on your team, someone with the common goal of all getting ahead together, but who also has a completely different skillset and advantage to you – just as you have a completely different advantage to her. You are shaped uniquely. She is, too. When you understand this, you'll be comfortable with her succeeding, because you'll realise you *both* succeed when one of you is.'

'Yeah, I do get that, but I'm sick of never being the one to do very well. I'm a fucking joke, Bro. I always have been.'

'Bro! Do you ever stop to think how she must see you? She married you! An amazing, intelligent woman married you. She must see something that you're missing!'

I felt bad that he truly didn't think he offered much, and I wanted to encourage him.

'Honestly, Bro. The fact that you persist and keep going shows me what you're made of. It's easy to do things in life we love and are naturally good at. It takes a great deal of perseverance to keep showing up when we aren't the best at something. For every person coming first in a race there's a lot more in the same race not getting a placing. Should they just not bother?'

At that he looked up. 'I just want to be the best at one thing, Bro! One thing! Is that honestly too much to ask?'

'No, my Bro, but you are *already* the best at one thing – and it's the one thing that matters. You just don't see it. You are a really good Dad to Lenny. Honestly, I've always admired that about you. You are so present with her and make so much effort.

I'll never forget the birthday party you threw for her when your wifey was working. You did amazing, and I thought most Fathers in your position wouldn't have gone to the lengths you did. I probably wouldn't have! But honestly, she saw and appreciated every single detail. Every detail told her that she mattered, and that her Dad valued her so much because he went to this much effort. If you could only see what really matters, Bro. None of that other stuff matters. Forget making your Dad proud. You're making Lenny proud. You're being a better Father than you ever had, and by doing that you should be proud of yourself.'

We talked some more and hugged again. We had the kind of long hug that I knew meant he was in a better place in his mind.

I'VE HAD COUNTLESS MOMENTS like this with men over the years, and my favourite moments are when the truth hits them and drives out the delusions they've been living under. For me, there is nothing quite as exciting as when a truthful new insight hits them. I can physically see their perspective change. It's the only thing I've really ever seen work. It can literally change *everything* about how they see their life in a matter of seconds.

I'm not saying that ongoing work isn't needed to change mindsets and behaviour, because it is a daily task to align our mind with the truth, but the saying *'The truth shall set you free'* is what I have literally based my whole life and career on. Can I add that, yes, it sets you free – but first it stings a bit!

She was never my friend's competition. His wife had always been his teammate. He just hadn't realised he was playing against his own team for so long.

I don't believe in being in competition with other people. I've been asked countless times to enter hair competitions around the world, and I've never wanted to, so I haven't. That's not because I think I'm too good, nor that I'm scared of losing. Either way, I just think that it's all subjective. How is any competition really judged fairly and accurately? I've been a judge for hair art competitions, and it's really hard to determine a clear winner based purely on skill, so in the end you choose the one that captured you personally, which could come down to you liking the image they picked to draw on a head.

How do we deem anyone to be the best at something? Especially when the things that an individual has to overcome to get there vary so much. I don't really believe in serious competition with others, and here's why: my 'best work' on any given day will be different. I have days after getting no sleep (for a week, thanks to kids who don't sleep), and then I have days of feeling rested and rejuvenated. My output on those days differs greatly. I could be 'the best' one day, and far from 'the best' another day. Where is the starting point? In life, no one starts from exactly the same place ever. Some have two awesome parents; some have only one. Some may have none. Some are naturally talented in a certain area, and develop skills very early in life, while others discover later – through experiences and being adventurous – what their sweet spot is. There is no one path.

The decision about who is 'the best' or who wins usually comes down to someone's opinion: what their personal taste is and what they personally enjoy informs their decision. When kids get interviewed for top-rated schools, part of the process, besides any previous school results, is if the interviewer likes the applicant. And let's be honest: some people interview better than others. Some people's nerves get the better of them.

Even competing at the Olympics comes down to if you can afford the opportunity to go. The cost of being a professional Olympic athlete, over their lifetime of training and expenses, is calculated to be around the six-figure mark. So let's be realistic: you aren't necessarily 'the best in the world', but you are the best out of those in the world who could afford to compete.

Please don't mistake this for me diminishing anyone's achievements either, or for saying you can be complacent about your gifts, talents and abilities. I'm naturally a perfectionist. I love creativity, and I feel really inspired by so many sources to constantly push myself in every area of my life. But how can I really compete with anyone? Other people's achievements really only serve as inspiration for seeing what is possible and what can be achieved – not necessarily by me – but their success triggers the desire within me to be brave enough to keep going courageously down my own path. It shows me what is possible.

I have my own story and my own path. Not a soul alive has what I bring to the table; my own siblings have different experiences and feelings, even though we all lived in the same childhood home. We each have our gifts that, along with our stories, make us a beautiful offering to the world. I encourage you to be focused on this.

Others can inspire you, but you, my Brother, have something unique. Develop that.

How could anyone compare the work of Leonardo da Vinci and Michelangelo? I've been to France and Italy and seen some of their masterpieces with my own eyes. Although they were alive at the same time, and are both considered to be Renaissance masters responsible for creating some of the greatest artwork in existence, they, too, were once in direct competition with each other when they ended up being commissioned to paint a vast battle scene on the same wall of a palazzo in Florence, Italy. They met each other through a man named Giorgio Vasari, who was also a historian of the Renaissance period. He said that with this competition came paranoia and hatred. Michelangelo made it so clear that he didn't like Leonardo that he left for France to avoid him. Leonardo, too, made unkind comments in his notebooks about the quality of Michelangelo's painting.

In the end, it ended up being the wall that never was, and a loss to the entire world. If they had been put together to collaborate instead of competing, would that have changed the outcome?

Instead of competition, I have learnt to understand the huge value of collaboration and community. I've learnt that what is meant for me will come for me, and what isn't best for me will pass me by in favour of someone who is just right for that opportunity. There's enough opportunity for us all. In all the closest relationships I have ever had, including that with my wife, I have found that collaboration sets me up the best, to foster a deep and genuine connection.

Chapter seventeen

She is not your bank account

ONCE, I HAD A GUY come straight out of jail to work for me. I'm a huge believer that for someone to make a full rehabilitation from prison, someone else has to be willing to take a shot on him, give him a chance, and teach him a trade so that he can have a job he can enjoy and feel proud to do on the outside. *And* so he is able to provide an income for himself and his family. No job, and the chances of reoffending are pretty high.

This wasn't the first ex-inmate I'd taken on. I've had success in doing this before through the work Sarah and I do in prisons. This particular guy had started barbering inside, and I heard about him through a friend of a friend. I don't ever hire anyone based on talent. I just have to see that he wants a chance and an opportunity for a different life. I knew he was a Father, so that was a tick – he had someone to be motivated enough to change for.

But, actually, the reason I hired him was his partner. I don't think I have ever met a girl who wanted this chance for her man so badly. She had waited for him the entire time he was inside, and had even forged a relationship with his ex-partner so that things were good enough with her that when he got out he would be able to see his child. She had been faithful, patient and supportive, and when he finally came out, here she was ready and hoping that he would seize the opportunity of a new life with grateful, open arms.

After I gave him the opportunity of working with us, she wrote to me and thanked me profusely. She was so committed that she helped buy him the barber gear he needed. She would even let him use her car so he could get to the barbershop with no problems, while she would catch an Uber back and forth to her own work. Simply put, she removed every barrier to him fully integrating back into life on the outside that he could have, and she gave him every single thing she possibly could. She had her own children, and even with that responsibility she went above and beyond to provide him with all that he needed, in the hope that he would - at a minimum - keep the job, and be faithful to her and the life she was offering him on a silver platter.

'You treat money you didn't earn very differently from money you legitimately earn. Money you don't earn is "easy come, easy go" and, deep down inside, it makes you feel useless.'

However, within weeks he had days of calling in 'sick', but I would find out that it was the after-effects from partying - even though he had strict probation conditions that forbade the consumption of alcohol or drug use. He admitted to me that he had cheated on her while under the influence of substances, within weeks of being out.

And, inevitably, it all came to a screeching halt when he didn't show up one day, and she messaged me, telling me that he had been partying and had gone out of town with a gang that he had just joined. This was after explicit warnings from her that she would leave him if he went back to that life. I appreciated her honesty and knew it would have been hard for her to be honest with me, knowing that this would end his job with me, and therefore any chance he had of a barbering career, or a legitimate way of making a living.

I also immediately messaged him to remind him that if he had re-joined a gang he no longer had a job with me. One of the very few requirements I have when the guys join our team is that they break any gang affiliation or connection. You cannot live successfully in two worlds. What I offer in my shop is a completely opposite life, but with the similar traits of Brotherhood, family, belonging and loyalty that I know most of those guys desire from gang life so much.

I knew she was feeling low. Here was a girl who had literally been his bank account, his currency and his opportunity for a completely different life. I told her that, unfortunately, while she had offered him the world, he wasn't grown-up enough to even understand what she was offering.

It was his loss. He ended up losing her, losing his relationship, losing access to his child, and going back inside.

It saddened me to see a man who had every opportunity to change his narrative, but didn't. I felt saddest for his son, another casualty of a lifestyle that always takes more than it ever gives. And I felt deeply for a woman who had bankrolled a guy who had invested zero into his own rehabilitation.

So to my Brothers out there who use women like this one, with no thought to the cost to her, I want to remind you that she is not disposable, and what she gives you may not cost *you* anything, but it does not come for free. You might not be paying the bill – but she is.

Not a damn thing comes for free.

TO BE BRUTALLY HONEST with you, I truly do not believe that – short of a severe mental illness, a medical condition, or an accident that leaves you disabled – there is a single plausible excuse in this world why you shouldn't be contributing in some way to paying for your own existence. When I hear a grown-ass man whining about not liking a job, or making excuses as to why he can't keep a job, or even apply for a job, I want to seriously shake him. It's even worse to me when these grown men have dependent children who actually need him to get off his ass to provide for them.

Here's the key to it all, Brother. You take any job and you work – doing that job to the best of your abilities – showing up every single day, until you can find a job that you might like better. Adopt the attitude that anything can teach you something, and that even the discipline of showing up day after day is building your character. When you actually secure a new job that you like better, only then can you quit the other job – because *any* job is better than no job. Clean toilets, work pushing trolleys – but whatever you do, actually *do it* wholeheartedly – every single day. By practising a good work ethic, showing up every day and improving yourself – that's how you get ahead. That's how you build your self-esteem. By working hard, doing your best, and bringing your pay home for your family.

I'll tell you a well-known secret. You treat money you didn't earn very differently from money you legitimately earn. Money you don't earn is 'easy come, easy go', and, deep down inside, it makes you feel useless. Regardless of what anyone says, the person wearing the fast-food uniform, or the cleaner's uniform, or the factory worker's uniform is miles ahead of the guy 'too cool' to work. Personal pride in yourself starts when you take your existence seriously enough to actually work for your survival.

And before you scoff at 'those kinds of jobs', I'll tell you where 'those kinds of jobs' get you. People doing these jobs were the essential workers who have kept New Zealand (and the world) going during the Covid-19 pandemic. And these jobs can also change your life.

ONE OF OUR CLOSEST friends' parents came to New Zealand from Iran because of religious persecution. They came over with nothing, and barely spoke English. They owned nothing. They had no family here. Not once did they receive a government handout. No benefits. Nothing. They simply worked in whatever jobs they could. Nothing was below them. They struggled. They raised two children and they saved every last cent they could. They lived as simply as possible. Eventually they bought their own house, and they now also own a rental property. Currently her parents are in their fifties, and her Father still works in a factory that makes sausages, while her Mother works in a bakery.

Now the proud owners of *two* homes, and the parents of children with university degrees, they are living proof that a positive attitude and hard work in jobs many would think to be beneath them will get you ahead in life – more than doing nothing ever will.

DON'T EVER FOOL YOURSELF into thinking that laziness and apathy is an acceptable way to live. You aren't becoming a 'professional gamer' playing video games all day. Nor are you a 'rapper' if you sleep all day and party all night with your 'crew'. Until the things you are doing bring in a legitimate income, and pay your bills, or are building your knowledge and skillset (like studying or learning a trade) to eventually earn money, you aren't doing anything except wasting time. And worse is when you are wasting time at *her* expense while she works and pays *your* bills. If you are sleeping in her bed, using her power and water, and eating her food, you can and absolutely should contribute to those expenses.

I've met grown men who rely solely on their girlfriends, wives or Mothers for money, and I want to ask them why they are refusing to grow up. Growing up means being an adult. Being an adult means being responsible. Being responsible means we learn to do things out of necessity, including things we may not want to do or like to do.

I think back to a lesson Sarah was attempting to teach our teenage daughter. It was her first year of exams at high school, and our daughter's passion and love in life is not really academics. She's musically and creatively gifted, and that day she was complaining about two of her least-liked but compulsory subjects: maths and science. She didn't want to have to take them as subjects, and she certainly didn't want to spend a second longer than she had to studying them. She would moan to us regularly about having to do any work on these subjects.

I remember one conversation Sarah had with her in the kitchen, and I thought: '*Here* is the lesson that many adults have not learnt.'

Sarah asked Oceana why she hated these particular subjects, and she responded that she didn't enjoy them, and she couldn't grasp the information easily.

'Oh, so because it doesn't come *easy* for you, you don't like to do it?'

Oceana nodded her head. 'Yes, that's it,' she said. 'Music and art I enjoy doing, so I just want to do things that I enjoy and I'm good at. It's a waste of time doing things I hate and I'm not good at.'

Sarah laughed out loud at that point. 'Oh, so you always want to do things you like and are good at, but you want to avoid doing anything you dislike and are not good at?'

Our daughter looked exasperated at this point. '*Yes,* that's right. That's what I said!'

'Yeah, sorry sweetie, but that's not reality,' Sarah told her. 'Adult life is learning to sometimes do stuff we don't enjoy doing. It's also learning to get better at doing things we aren't naturally good at. It's showing up consistently, day after day, when we sometimes want to give up. Do you honestly think that Dad feels like going to work every single day, and standing on his feet for twelve hours straight, cutting man after man when it's hot and there's hair stuck to him?'

Oceana looked over at me. 'Yeah, but Dad likes being a barber, and he's good at it - right, Dad?'

'Yeah,' I said. 'I do mostly love being a barber, but there are moments I don't enjoy it at all. There are moments when I think I'd rather be at home sitting on my computer making music, but I push through because, right now, this is how I support our family. Me, standing on my feet all day, means that you and your

She is not your bank account

siblings live in this house, and have food to eat. Every single job you do in life will probably have moments you don't enjoy so much. You have to take the not-so-great moments with the great moments. That's just life.'

'Do you think anyone wants to be a parent every single day?' Sarah added. 'There are nights I just want sleep so bad, I'd love to clock out. I don't want to have to clean up shit or cook another meal. I don't want to have to pay taxes, or even do the grocery shopping. If you learn to work hard now, studying subjects you hate, if you actually give your best when it doesn't come easily to you – that is character-building.'

'Great,' Oceana groaned loudly. 'It's one of *those* talks! All I said was that I hate science!'

We all ended up laughing and ended our lecture with: 'If you have the kind of character that means you will always show up, and consistently give your best – regardless of what job it is – you are the person who will out-work the person who only wants to do what's easy for them.'

After that speech, Oceana worked hard all year and passed both science and maths. We were so proud of her efforts, and we hope our daughter has grasped a bigger lesson for life. It's an important one to learn that seems to be hugely missing in many adults I meet as an employer.

MEN WHO REFUSE TO grow up and take financial responsibility for themselves stay stuck in the thinking that someone else will always pay the bill, cover the debt, and bail them out. They are the kind of guys who as grown adults think that their Mothers really like giving them money, but they don't check to see if their Mothers have eaten this week. They make their financial crises someone else's problem, and they expect to be rescued from their own bad relationship with money.

If you know you have a bad relationship with money, it's okay (again!) to ask for help. There are numerous organisations all over the world that offer free budgeting advice and support. They are confidential and non-judgemental, and can help you look at your debts and your income, and make a plan to turn poor money management around. You don't have to do this alone, but you do have to take the first step, because no one else can do that for you.

She is not your Bank Account, and she owes you nothing.

But if you take ownership of your finances, she can be your business partner - someone who grows the empire of your life with you. And it's for this reason that, when I'm speaking at a high school or a youth group about entrepreneurial life, I make sure I paint an accurate picture - and I do this because barbering gave me this life. Not hustling, not gang life, not my parents giving me handouts, or me living off my wife. The long days and nights barbering in a tin garden shed in the hood started building my empire.

'My parents had never received any handouts throughout their lives. They had multiple low-paying jobs, and as I grew up I knew that if I wanted something it was, indeed, up to me.'

There were no shortcuts, grants or loans. I have never borrowed money from anyone for my business - not the bank nor my family. No one gave me a cent, and when I had outgrown the tin shed in the hood, I wondered how I would get the money required for a deposit and the fit-out of a proper barbershop. Sarah was clear and very direct with me: 'No one will lend you a cent. You have no credit history, and you own nothing. We'll have to find ways to make the money ourselves.'

So we did.

And after touring and delivering our barbering education tutorials all over New Zealand and Australia, in the space of a few months we had enough money to be able to open our first barbershop on one of the busiest streets in Christchurch. Every cent that it cost came from our hard work, and it felt good.

The night before we opened the new barbershop, I walked outside and looked at it. A handful of Brothers had helped us by investing hours of their labour in building and painting to get it looking great. I'll forever be thankful for their investment and will never forget it. Sarah was pregnant with our son, and we stood there, hand in hand, and marvelled at what we had accomplished together.

And finally, on the chilly night of our grand opening in August 2014, our entire community came to support us and bear witness to the fruition of a dream that a Sāmoan kid from the hood had. I had grown up with very little materially, but I had seen the work ethic that my parents lived by, and while they had many shortcomings, their work ethic was always second to none.

My parents had never received any handouts throughout their lives. They had multiple low-paying jobs, and as I grew up I knew that if I wanted something it was, indeed, up to me.

On opening night, as I gave my speech to those attending, and looked over at Sarah, I saw in her the partner I wanted – someone to dream and make plans with. She was someone I could work alongside, and build our empire together. I knew she had my back – as I had hers – and if she hadn't specifically told me that I was *not* to propose to her in the barbershop, I probably would have, right there in that moment.

Because I knew then, with no doubt at all, she was the 'ride-or-die girl' for me. She equalled me in the relationship. Neither was there to bankroll the other.

We both came with the mindset to contribute our best – and it is with this mindset that we have built our entire relationship, business and lifestyle. We built a partnership that was based on us each bringing our best to the table, and working together with what we have. And it's been *this* foundation on which everything we've built since has been based. When I am regularly asked for business advice I will say: 'Start with what you have, where you are.' Because the truth is that's all we ever really have, and it's a solid foundation on which to grow a life of substance.

Chapter eighteen

She is not your quick fix

FIRST UP, MY DISCLAIMER is that I - 100% - do not believe there is an actual quick fix for anything.

Not weight loss.

Not mental health issues.

Not relationship problems.

Not financial problems.

Not addictions.

Not violence.

If it seems too good to be true, then it usually is.

Unless you do the consistent work required - the work that brings changes that can last you a lifetime - then it's a quick fix. Quick fixes do not ever work long term.

All of the issues listed above are simply behaviours that outwardly indicate that you have a deeper issue, and it's usually because of a subconscious and untrue belief that you are loyal to. Or it's a survival kit that worked for you when you were younger, to protect you from some kind of childhood trauma, but doesn't work at all now as an adult. What it's actually doing is destroying the life you really want.

What it all means is that you have work to do, and by work I do mean hard, uncomfortable - but ultimately rewarding - work. You are going to have to find the lie you have told yourself is true and then tell yourself a new truth. Does that sound easy? It's not. It requires a long-term commitment from you to identify and change beliefs and behaviour that, by now, come as second nature.

I'm someone who has struggled with my weight my entire adult life, and it's still something that I have to work on. To be honest, it's something I will probably have to work on for the rest of my life. First of all, I have a Polynesian build. We aren't really a small people to begin with. Secondly, I love food - and because of this I seem to gain weight so easily. Basically, if I see fried chicken it jumps on my hips almost as soon as it touches my lips!

Food is a huge part of our culture. All of our family and cultural gatherings include food. This is good-tasting food that is not low in carbohydrates or calories. My Father also has some Chinese heritage, but unfortunately none of his children inherited his lithe Asian build. We all take after my Mother's side - we are all solid, with a tendency to put weight on quickly.

My youngest brother Nu is a professional athlete and plays rugby league internationally, so it's his job to stay in shape. Whenever he gets his few weeks off each year to come home and be with his family, he eats all the food he wants to that he's usually not allowed, and he stacks on the weight by about a kilo a day. That's the kind of food we love.

Luckily for him, he goes back to his life and immediately goes back onto his eating regime and exercise schedule, which enables him to quickly shed the excess kilograms. The rest of us are not paid to stay in shape, so trust me, we don't make the same effort, nor give it the priority that he does, to burn it off.

I've been successful with various diets before. The ones I like the best were where I could drop about 5 kilograms a week, which was great for occasions such as a wedding or a trip, but I know that - unless it's a lifestyle change I'm willing to implement for the rest of my life - the weight just creeps back on. Actually, who am I kidding? My weight *runs* back on the second I see a burger!

I share this with you because I would say it's probably been one of the biggest struggles of my life. I started struggling with it after I was sexually abused in my adolescent years. Food was a comfort and a reliable friend, and somehow this – mixed with nutritionally bad (but tasty) food choices, eating large portions, or eating whatever was available at home at irregular times – meant that by the time I left home I was already well over the 'recommended weight' for my height.

Fast-forward to married life, and my wife is a great cook who makes beautiful meals and delicious food that is good for us, but still I eat portions that, really, are too big for what I require, and I still like snacking at night if I'm working late. All this, mixed with a lack of exercise and not the best sleeping patterns (thanks, kids!), and you have a guy who is much heavier than he needs to be.

'There's a major problem when you expect your partner to fulfil every role in your life, instead of stepping into that role yourself. I've learnt for myself that no one soul can ever be everything to us. We all need a community or a village of people around us who serve different purposes.'

In moments of being on my latest fad diet, I have expected Sarah to make specially prepped containers of on-the-go meals ready for my consumption. If she's been too busy, I've actually found myself blaming her for me not losing weight – even though I could easily make the meals myself. It's easier to expect someone else to solve our issues and make them magically go away, because if they fail us then it's now their fault.

My wife sees through my bullshit like she has a radar detector for it. Immediately she calls me to account. 'If you want specially prepared meals that I don't have the time to make, you will have to make them yourself, or take responsibility for failing at your eating plan. Your weight loss is not my responsibility,' she says.

Touché! Point taken, and this leads me to wonder how much of our unsuccessful attempts at overcoming addictions or issues do we blame on others, simply because that is easier than taking responsibility for it ourselves?

There really are no shortcuts to wholeness and healing, or even success. Most of us would say we'd like to win Lotto, or at least have the permanent financial freedom to live the life we really desire. Yet how many of us are actually prepared to make the consistent daily choices, and the sacrifices, wise decisions and investments needed to be in the position of wealth? We just want the end result, without putting the work into getting it. Consider the fact that a high percentage of lottery winners lose their entire winnings within a year of hitting the jackpot, because they simply don't know how to keep it. They didn't go through the work of slowly building it up, so it slips through their fingers.

It's like that with anything. She cannot be something you use temporarily to suddenly skip over an issue that needs work. Just like a Lotto win is a quick fix to a person who isn't good with their finances, likewise a person who hopes their partner will be a quick fix for whatever addiction or suffering they are going through will be disappointed when the cracks begin to show. They haven't done the work to find the core issues that need to be resolved before they can have long-term healing.

As a matter of fact, she is not your therapist, your entertainment director, your shrink, your trainer or even your counsellor. It is *not* her sole responsibility to make sure you are living the life you want. You don't get to demand that she orchestrate it all, and make it magically happen for you.

Think of therapy like dental hygiene: it only really works if you do it regularly enough to make your teeth healthy, and it requires ongoing maintenance. Your teeth are always changing, and your dental professional will pick up on those changes. If you have a deeper issue like a root canal, then just brushing your teeth occasionally won't do anything. If you leave it, you'll just be in pain for longer, and it will cost more to fix in the long run.

You may need to work regularly with a professional therapist to gently uncover the emotional issues you have. This may take several sessions, but it is worth doing the work. A token session here and there is barely going to scratch the surface - you need to commit to doing this for yourself. It's your pathway to healing.

My journey with therapy has really opened my eyes to things I've struggled with. I couldn't have worked through my pornography addiction without professional help. I couldn't have learned new ways of thinking and rewired my brain without professional help. And every wānanga and workshop that Sarah and I facilitate offers a different kind of therapy to the men we work alongside, and shows me just how much support is needed for lasting change.

Through this journey, I have realised:

My happiness isn't up to her.

The fulfilment of my dreams isn't up to her.

My health isn't up to her.

My career success isn't up to her.

I'm not her project.

My life is not her job to 'fix'.

Nor is she 'the reason' why I am not where I want to be.

SARAH IS NOT RESPONSIBLE for *any* part of my life more than I am.

There is a famous saying: 'The buck stops with me.' It refers to the notion that we have to make decisions and then accept the ultimate responsibility for those decisions and their consequences.

Taking ownership of your life decisions is probably the single most empowering thing you can do for yourself. You are now saying 'This is my life, and I choose - in every aspect - the way that I live it', because genuine growth and healing mean you actually have to get real with yourself about the role you play in your own suffering.

And while it might be nice, in theory, to have someone who makes sure our life's goals are their priority to accomplish, it also comes at a cost to the woman/partner in your life. If she's so busy helping you to achieve your goals, when does she have time to work on hers? In our relationship, I also want to see Sarah accomplishing her goals and feeling validated. My success cannot come at the cost of hers.

I have met men who, out of some strange thinking, blame their wife or partner for them not being where they want to be, and sometimes I stand back and listen to their excuses.

Take Dave, for example. I've known him since before he was married. They were married over a decade, and he and his wife have beautiful children together. He appeared to have a successful career in a high-profile job, but he was still not happy with his life. Not only did he compare himself to the other, more successful men around him, but he also compared his wife to other wives.

One day, we were talking about his life and his marriage. He had been unhappy for a while, and I asked him: 'Dave, what do you really want from your wife?'

'To either get on board, and help me make our lives happen, or move the hell over and let me be free to make it happen by myself.' He said it so quickly, and in such a matter-of-fact way, that it was obvious he had been thinking about this for a while.

'What if she lets you go, and you still don't make your dreams come true?' I asked.

'It won't happen,' he said. 'Honestly, if you knew the calibre of women who hit me up, you'd understand, Bro. They're the go-getters in life, and, as much as I love my wife, she's not that. I thought she'd be more help once the kids were older, but it's a no-go. She's just not inclined that way.'

'Right,' I thought. 'Clearly the same calibre of women who would hit on a married man.' I shook my head.

Dave's wife is sweet, kind and a great Mother. She takes pride in parenting their children lovingly, and is the most present Mother you could ever want for your children. She's also the most encouraging and loyal wife imaginable. She's someone who could be happy living simply, just as long as her family was together and okay, because she is not really very materialistic. She is someone who is not ambitious either. She's not lazy, and she works part-time in a job she enjoys, but she genuinely doesn't care about material things in the way that Dave does, and clearly that's a sore point for him.

They married young, and initially everything seemed fine. They both had a sincere love and loyalty for each other and their family. They had similar morals and values to begin with, but 10 years down the track he expected to be further along in life. He wanted the big house and more money, and he blamed her for their not being at that point. Her lack of interest in having the things he believed would make them happy meant that they were never in agreement.

In his eyes, the attributes he had once considered beautiful had become the very things now holding him back. To him, her lack of material ambition was a very plausible reason why they weren't where he deemed they should be. She wasn't 'fixing' his problems at all.

It also came down to priorities. For her, they were being present for their children, and it was most important to have family time and connection. His priority was having things. I asked him one day if he was grateful for what he did have – a loving, loyal wife, beautiful children, and a well-paid job that gave them a comfortable life.

He looked me square in the eye and said: 'It's just not enough for me. I love my wife, and yes, she's a good woman – and I love my kids, too. But they're getting in the way of the things I really want in life. They're a bit of a hindrance, really.'

I was shocked to hear it put so bluntly. From the outside looking in, this guy really had the good life, and I knew a long line of men who would happily have traded places with him.

'Honestly, Bro,' I said, 'you might think that is what you really want, but a woman like your wife is hard to find, trust me. If you're both so ambitious and focused on this insatiable goal of yours, who is raising your kids? You've always told me that family life is so important to you, but what kind of family life is it if both parents are so focused on making money and acquiring stuff? Your children grow up fast, and this time you have with them is precious. The fact that your wife is focusing on them now is not a bad thing.'

'Bro, honestly – she's holding me back, and not supporting my vision in the way I need her to. I know I'm not happy, and I know I can find someone better,' he insisted.

With that the conversation was over, and eventually his marriage was, too. I can't help but think he would have been much better off if he just hired a life coach or a financial advisor to give him some guidance to help him set his personal goals, without expecting her to fix it all.

THERE'S A MAJOR PROBLEM when you expect your partner to fulfil every role in your life, instead of stepping into that role yourself. I've learnt for myself that no one soul can ever be everything to us. We all need a community or a village of people around us who serve different purposes. My wife is a great all-rounder, but I have male friends who I unwind with, or sometimes debrief with over a coffee or a whisky. These conversations are gifts.

Sometimes we, as men, have emotions that are best understood and talked over with other men. I've always been mindful to not just dump all my garbage on my wife like she's a rubbish dump, because that emotional labour shouldn't be expected of her – or of any woman. Why should she have to sort through all my crap, when I haven't taken the time to sort through it myself?

We have to be careful of hurting those we love because we haven't done the work on our unhealed emotions. We need to be able to identify our own emotions first, and be able to sit with our triggers before we can talk about them. Often those emotions have nothing to do with our wives or partners – they're from old hurts and pain. It's unfair to expect her to fix those, too.

I've been mindful of selecting good guys who not only listen to what I'm saying, but who also offer insight and objectivity. This is insight gained from experience, and lessons learnt personally, and the kind of insight that sometimes only comes from someone who is outside the situation. Often, when we are stuck in a confusing or overwhelming situation, they are the ones who see things clearly. It's in these conversations that I have learnt that often feelings are not facts, and we sometimes need to verbally debrief with someone who has a different perspective to get to the core issue.

'I absolutely believe there is a right time for all of us. Sometimes we just have to grow into the right person for this opportunity to find us at the right time.'

My advice to you all is to have one or two trusted guys who you can do this with. Other men who have your best interests at heart, and who are good at listening and really hearing you. It's worth holding onto a good barber who can do this with you, too, because in this current 'busy' generation it is not uncommon for me to meet men who have no other men they can really talk with, and who also have very little encouragement in their lives. My clients have shared things with me that their own families don't know. Most of the time he doesn't even want advice, he just wants to be heard. Brother, let me also say here that the same thing applies to your wife or partner. Sometimes she doesn't want you to solve her problems either, but just to listen to her.

Often you'll find that just being heard offers you the clarity that you don't get when you are lost and alone in your thoughts.

There are also things that are obviously best discussed with experts in their field - therapists, counsellors and professional support people. There are times when - despite our very best intentions and desires - we just can't seem to get to where we want to be. This could be with your mental or physical health, your emotional wellbeing, or even your career.

If you are feeling stuck for a prolonged period in your life, then trust me when I say there *is* someone out there who can help you, and - thankfully - we now live in an age where everything is accessible at the touch of your fingertips. We have to understand and really comprehend that the power to change any part of our lives is up to us, and starts with us taking the initiative to find someone in the particular area we need help in to assist us with the right tools, or point us to the right book or podcast.

I BELIEVE ALSO THAT we have to grasp the idea that in life there are seasons for everything. I've had seasons where there seem to be endless challenges coming at me, and very little movement. It was hugely frustrating, and it wasn't until I was further down the track that I realised that that season of challenge where I'd felt stagnant was actually a season of great learning and growth that I needed to experience before the next season of opportunity came.

We are not always ready for what we want when we first want it. Doing the work to get to where we want to be will not always be as quick or as easy as we want or expect it to be. Achieving something is never a quick or easy fix.

And, other than finding a life coach or therapist to assist you to achieve your goals, or find the right insight, the biggest piece of advice I can offer is to make peace with who you are, and where you are, at any given moment of life. Sometimes the moment we make peace with where we are is the moment we move.

Sometimes we have to make peace with our success not being in the timeline we wanted. Time will no longer be your enemy if you can grasp these concepts, because we're all so uniquely shaped, with our own paths and experiences. Don't bother comparing yourself with someone else, because it really is a waste of time. Over time I have learnt that the great voids we feel in between the moments of 'grinding' and 'success' are all a necessary part of life.

Music has always been my first passion. From the time I was

a child, the most consistent dream I've ever had was to be a teacher or to do something musically. It was all I ever wanted to be, and I have always known that, in due time, the deepest desire of my heart would somehow come into fruition. I left home when I was 15 to support myself into adulthood. This meant I turned down an arts scholarship in order to start a trade in joinery so I could earn money to support myself. I spent years overcoming childhood trauma, and for a number of years I was purely in survival mode – there was no time for dreams or following artistic pursuits.

No one will ever know or understand the energy that is required to raise yourself unless you've spent that energy yourself. At the end of every day there isn't much left, so any dreams you dare to have are drip-fed slowly, whenever possible. But more often than not, it isn't possible to work on your dreams consistently.

Years passed. I kept living that same monotonous cycle:

Wake up.

Go off to work at a job that paid my bills but didn't feed my soul.

Go back home to eat.

Watch something on TV.

Sleep.

Repeat.

However, I believe that Atua (or God, as I understand Him to be) had a plan for me, and eventually made way for what seemed so impossible to me for years.

I absolutely believe there is a right time for all of us. Sometimes we just have to grow into the right person for this opportunity to find us at the right time. Make no mistake: you are not forgotten or overlooked. How can you be, when you are the only living person able to do what you do in this world?

Be ready in anticipation for that moment. The doors of opportunity will present themselves, and, when they open, it will be time to walk right through. Are you really ready for that? If success is when preparation meets opportunity, then ask yourself, how prepared are you for opportunity to arrive?

If you aren't ready, then start to get ready. Stay fertile in your thinking. By that I mean: align yourself with the truth of who you are in all moments. Be honest about your strengths and shortcomings. Ask yourself, what areas can you improve in? Align yourself with people who tell you the truth and genuinely support your growth. It's okay to be in what seems to be a stagnant season, but trust that this isn't going to last and that maybe there is something you need to learn so that you can move from the void to opportunity.

You don't need to rush your growth, though, Brother. You want growth to come from an authentic place of knowledge that you have gained through your own experiences. Look for the insight and be prepared for the lesson, because our lessons and our insights are as unique as we are, and they will come when we are ready. It may seem to be a cliché, but **what we seek we do inevitably find.**

In all our collective quick fixes, I wonder if we can stop and examine what is happening long enough to see that all our quick fixes, and our survival kits - all our ways of coping - are just us acknowledging there is pain within ourselves that we are trying so hard to manage/control/hide/not feel.

And the question really is: **Will we have the courage to go deeper?**

Go deeper, beyond the excuses, to the reason why we aren't where we want to be.

That place is where we begin to heal.

Chapter nineteen

She is not your trophy

IF YOU HAPPEN TO view the woman in your life as *'a decorative object awarded as a prize for a victory or success'*, then this chapter is for you.

The story I'm about to tell you may seem pretty extreme, but, at the heart of it, it is actually really common, and I see it regularly. People who see their association or relationship with other people as a way to make themselves appear cooler, better, more attractive, worthier, more interesting, more cultured, wealthier, more intelligent or even more successful.

Many years ago, Sarah worked in a beauty salon. It was in quite an affluent area, and attracted a well-heeled clientele who had the money to enjoy being pampered. They had one rather memorable client who was in her twenties, and married to a very wealthy man who was in his late fifties. He was extremely loud, with a demanding, abrasive and obnoxious personality. Without fail, he would come into the salon with his wife and explain to the nail technician exactly how he wanted her nails done. She was allowed two tanning sessions each month to maintain what he said was the perfect colour. 'Not too dark, but looking like the sun kissed her and left a golden glow,' he stipulated.

Not only did he do this here, but also at the nearby hair salon where her bleached blonde hair was regularly touched up. She'd also had multiple plastic surgery procedures at his request, and had to maintain a very specific weight. This specific weight included the provision that she was never to have children, because he didn't want her to ruin her perfect figure. Thanks to all this work she was extremely attractive, and wore the latest designer outfits which he carefully picked out. It was her full-time job to look good for him.

Sarah noticed that there was something a little sad and slightly insecure about her, and asked the long-serving nail technicians more about their story. Apparently, he had been married before, and his first wife and children had left him, causing great humiliation. *'Who is she to leave me?'* he had been quoted as saying. Clearly his pride had taken a hit.

One of the staff had commented that he would have been better off to marry a mannequin with no thoughts and feelings of her own, because he was the main star of the show and his wife was an extra, merely there to make the scene more visually appealing.

Following a somewhat ugly divorce, he met his young wife and took over her life in every sense. He took her to every social occasion and party in the vicinity, as if to flaunt her beauty in a bid to gain some kind of new credibility following the divorce. She was known as his arm candy, his prize, and then as his trophy wife, as she dutifully tagged along with him and a much older crowd. Little was known about her except that she had no real family, and had few friends outside of him and his circle.

Her very existence was a mere extension of him.

Sarah said when you saw them together it was like seeing Beauty and the Beast – but not like the fairy tale. Sadly, it was obvious to all that his most attractive feature was, unfortunately, his massive bank balance. Her attractiveness didn't enhance his appearance, and her sweet, obliging personality didn't make his demanding personality any more palatable. As Sarah says: 'You can't put icing on bullshit and call it a cupcake!'

I know men who not only want their wives to look and be a certain kind of way, even down to the length of their hair, but they'll try to pick friends for this reason, too. They also believe that their children are an extension of themselves, and will put some pretty specific criteria on them to conform to the expectations they have – including who they can be friends with and what kind of interests they can have.

This controlling behaviour is not love. This is quite simply 'persuading' someone to come around to your way of thinking, because otherwise you'll make their lives difficult with your passive-aggressive comments, your angry outbursts, or the silent treatment you give them. And all this demonstrates is that you getting your way matters more to you than any opinion or desire she may have of her own.

'All the accolades, trophies, awards and praise in the world just don't compensate for the lack we can feel within us from not feeling adequate or worthy.'

The truth is that no other living, breathing soul is an extension of us. Not our wives, not our friends or family, and not even our children. 'By association' doesn't make you anything other than who you really are. If I hang around with doctors, that doesn't give me a medical degree. I have never agreed with the 'fake it till you make it' philosophy when it comes to having real relationships. **You can only be loved as much as you are truly known.** And to do this **you have to be free to be exactly who you are**, and then others will either love you as you are, or not really love you at all. And the same goes for your partner.

To consider her as your trophy is to care more about your status and how other people perceive *you* than actually valuing a genuine connection and a relationship based on who she is, rather than how she looks.

Many men are very deliberate in seeking out 'Trophies' in life to validate their worth, and to prove tangibly to others who they are, and their ability to acquire what they deem to be symbols of success. These men unashamedly use their Trophies to bring them the attention and accolades they feel they might not be able to attain just by themselves.

The media regularly feed us ideals of what a 'perfect' life looks like, and there seems to be a lot of pressure to attain those things - looking the 'right' (skinny) way, living in the 'right' neighbourhood, sending the kids to the 'right' schools with the 'right' friends, earning a massive six- or seven-figure salary, and driving the right cars. And if we don't live that kind of life, somehow we're failures.

Don't get me wrong. There's nothing wrong with acquiring assets or enjoying nice things. But things are really just things.

Are things all you think your life is worth? Are you just playing a part and living out a visual fantasy that society tells you represents success? This version of success doesn't actually guarantee genuine love, peace, joy, contentment or belonging. It's an insecure and fearful man who doesn't have the courage to live the life he really wants to live, regardless of what anyone else thinks.

Do you really want to go through your life ticking boxes, acquiring assets you give more meaning to than they deserve, and collecting women like inanimate objects? Making a woman into a trophy dehumanises her, as it systematically devalues her and undermines her from ever being considered your equal. Instead, she becomes something to own and to conquer.

There will always be another trophy - another model or a newer, upgraded version. We're urged to spend more, and want more, when what we really need to do is to *be* more. We need to work on the ultimate indicator of who we really are and what we are really about. Our **character**.

Your character is really the 'trophy' that will be remembered the most by anyone who knew you, when your time on this Earth comes to an end. This is the trophy of your life that also depends solely on you – regardless of your circumstances.

Your character dictates how you treat your wife/partner/girlfriend when no one else is around. I've met plenty of men whose workmates' version of them is very different to their wives' version of who they are. Your character determines if you are the same person in all situations.

Your character actually dictates how you treat women in general. Are you someone who advocates for women in your workplace or your church, or do you still believe they should be kept subdued and subjugated? Or do they need to be put on a pedestal, and admired from afar?

Your character dictates whether you laugh at the crass jokes with 'the boys' that demean and disrespect women. Is it really that funny to make an inappropriate joke at her expense? How do you think it makes her feel?

Your character dictates whether you are someone to be trusted with women you are not in a relationship with.

Your character dictates whether people feel safe with you. Are you someone who women or children feel comfortable around alone?

Your character dictates whether your physical or eye contact with women is inappropriate or lingers way too long. There are always the men whose very presence feels uncomfortable and 'off' because he does not respect her space and refuses to adhere to her boundaries. Women pick up on this immediately and try to avoid these 'space-invaders' like the plague. We all know that unfortunately men like this exist everywhere – in workplaces, at social gatherings and, unfortunately, even in our own families. Do you really want to be the guy that women actively avoid?

Your character determines what you prioritise in your life – what you give your energy to and for. Are you the family man or the playboy? Are you loyal to your wife in every sense of the word, or do you think it's okay to flirt with others? How important is it that she feels secure in your relationship with her? Does the loyalty you expect from her match the loyalty you give her?

All the accolades, trophies, awards and praise in the world can't compensate for the lack we can feel within us from not feeling adequate or worthy. Things will never bring fulfilment, and the most beautiful woman on your arm will never do the work you need to do for yourself to discover and understand your intrinsic worth.

You are loved and are lovable. You deserve to be here. You deserve to be in a relationship with someone who wholeheartedly chooses you – not for what you can do for them, but simply for who you are.

Who you are is dependent on you and the work you are prepared to do.

Do you come from a wounded place that still requires healing, or do you come from a scarred place that once survived trauma, but has healed from it? Brothers – there is a huge difference. A wound versus a scar.

In your daily life, when you interact with those around you, where do *you* come from? A wounded man is one in pain. A scarred man is one whose scar doesn't inflict him with the pain that his wound once did. The difference between the two is simple: it is healing.

Will you allow yourself to heal?

Think about when you are in physical pain from an injury – it may have been from a sports game, or an accident, or even a surgery. Are you in the best position to go about your typical work or daily tasks? Of course not. Most of us will give ourselves a break and allow time for recovery, yet many of us do not allow ourselves the same grace when it comes to emotional healing.

If we are looking outside ourselves – to someone or something to give us validation or meaning – that's a really good indicator that inner work is required.

When I think of the character of men I personally know and greatly admire, without fail they have a solid, honest relationship with a woman of their equal. In many ways she refines his character.

I think of my friend Kenyon. He's an extremely successful

property developer, and he's done extraordinarily well in life. Now in his early forties, he's smart, driven, drives a Ferrari or a Rolls Royce (depending on the day), lives in a big house with great views, has four beautiful children who go to the best schools, and anyone could look in at his life from the outside and define him as successful by society's standards. Over his lifetime he's lost millions and earned millions back again, and has done so with transparency by prioritising the relationships in his life.

Now having said all this, I'm not someone who measures success in life with just those material indicators, because that, to me, shows success in only one part of life. In my opinion, you are truly successful only if the people closest to you genuinely like you, because they actually know you, and you feel comfortable to be yourself – the same person – everywhere. So Kenyon needed a little more than that to score the points.

In most of the social situations I find myself in, I'm an observer, and when I first met Kenyon I remember sitting in his house listening to him talk. Our wives went to high school together, and have been friends for more than 20 years. Here is this guy who lives in a completely different world from me, sharing space with me, and I was fascinated by how his mind worked. He moves in completely different circles from me, and we have many differing views and experiences of life. But I thought to myself then, at our very first meeting: 'This guy deeply loves his wife and his family.' I could see he genuinely respected her and valued what she had to say. This has always stuck with me, and when I picture him this is what I see. Not the bling and the fancy things.

I've been in plenty of social settings where I've heard men blatantly disregard their wives, arrogantly dismissing or belittling them in public. That tells me more about their own insecurity, so it's a joy when I see a man stand in his own confidence, brilliance and mana, and still be a good guy because he isn't a slave to his ego.

It was refreshing watching them interact. Even when Kenyon and Charlotte would openly disagree with each other in front of other people, it was always done respectfully. Both could maintain their sense of self, have their own opinions, and share these with each other without any fear. I admired how he listened to her intently, taking her views seriously, even when he may not have shared similar views or ideas, and I especially admired when he could admit he was wrong, too. He was open to her knowing more than him, or even having a better idea about something.

She gave him the same respect, and I loved how they could also amicably agree to disagree and move on from a subject, or meet in the middle to find a solution. I saw the way he honoured her at a fundraising event they hosted for their charity foundation. He genuinely admired her, and he wanted the room to know.

I could see that this smart, attractive lady was far more than a trophy wife – she was his partner. This strong, successful man had a true partner in his wife because she was his equal. She was his equal because what she contributed to their life and business was valued immensely and mattered to him. Her views and thoughts were of no threat to him, and sharpened or balanced his own, and she knew that, and was secure in what she brought to the table.

In essence, they refined each other's character.

What a beautiful place to be. Are you up for that? It's time to step up and seek an equal partner. Are you ready to level up?

Chapter twenty

She is not your grief

I WRITE THIS CHAPTER in grief.

I write this because I am not immune to grief. None of us are. Grief is part of this journey of humanity.

My beloved Mother left this world as I was finishing this book, after being diagnosed with terminal lung cancer only four months prior. So I write this as a man who, on my birthday, went and knelt at her grave and sobbed loudly into the dirt that I miss her. Because I do, and I always will.

This is okay. My tears are acceptable. My grief is understandable.

Part of my grief is my sincere apology for all the times I fell short in being her son, wishing and longing that her life was better and that somehow I could have made it better, but knowing I didn't. Grief for me is not only the cost of loving her the way I did, but also the pain of the regret that our story and our trauma at times barricaded away the closeness I feel we deserved.

I write this as a man who, just a few weeks later, found out that my beloved day-one client, who has come to me from when I was cutting boys in my hood in my tin-shed barbershop in the garden, who has become a close Brother to me, is also now terminally ill with cancer, and does not have long to go before he departs this Earth, leaving behind a wife and three beautiful daughters.

When I think of the men I feel called to in this work of inviting men to heal, I firstly and always think of him, and how honoured I am that he bravely took down his walls and allowed me into his heart. Allowing me in meant I got to see him, and know him, and therefore love him. What a precious gift - and yet now my grief is the cost. A cost I would pay a thousand times over for having been able to know him the way I have.

I write about grief from this, a place of deep grief and genuine desire that death was not part of the experience of living. Yet it is, so in my own place of loss I write from a place of pain and reluctant acceptance.

Because I don't believe the devastation of losing a soul we love ever really leaves. Maybe we learn to live with it, but, regardless, if this is your pain, my Brother, then my heart is right here aching with you.

Without doubt, losing one of my children is my biggest fear in life. I think this is because we can anticipate there is a possibility that some people will go before us, like my Mother, my Grandparents and Aunties or Uncles have. The simple fact of them being older than me has meant their loss in my lifetime was expected at some point. That's not to say it's not painful, because losing my Mother has been indescribable agony in such a profound way. Even though I knew she was passing once she was diagnosed as terminal, there was still no way to prepare for her passing, and for the inevitable avalanche of emotions and grief that came from losing her; the woman I owe my life to.

And in feeling the way I do burying my Mother, I keep coming back to wondering how any parent recovers after burying their own child. You expect them to bury you - not the other way around. It seems like the direction of the circle of life has been broken when this occurs. Like you were ripped off from the life that was meant to be.

And it is this grief - the grief of the deep pain from the loss of a child - that I want to address with you here. Because it was a tsunami of grief that completely destroyed Gareth, a man who didn't ever recover when his daughter tragically drowned. When she drowned, so, in a way, did he.

Grief is a response to loss. That could be any kind of loss, but in Gareth's case it was the death of his daughter that plunged him into grief, and he's stayed there for more than 20 years. Ultimately, his inability to process his grief has cost him his marriage, and his relationship with his remaining children.

Gareth was a proud Father. His ex-wife says he was born to be a Father, and he was hands-on from day one. He would take their newborn baby off in his truck to drive around and show his construction clients. Gareth and his wife were best friends, and worked hard together in their business.

Their daughter wasn't quite two when she accidentally drowned on their property.

'It was no one's fault, but I think he blamed himself for not watching her in that moment, and he couldn't live with himself and with the reality that she was gone,' Gareth's wife told me.

The next morning, he was lying in bed, and he said to his wife, with eyes full of sorrow: 'I'm scared to get out of bed.'

He was scared to feel the grief that was overwhelming him. It took over their lives, and it manifested in different ways. For Gareth, it manifested firstly in anger and rage, and then in shame.

'The night after the funeral, it was just us at home. We had a disagreement about the music we were listening to, and he angrily stormed out of the room. I followed after him, and begged him to come back. I reached out to touch his arm, and he ended up throwing me against the wall, splitting open my face. He hadn't done anything like that before, so I excused it as an after-effect of shock. It was the first time I had seen anger like that from him. It was a far cry from the man I fell in love with. He had never ever even raised his voice to me before.'

Not only were they grappling with their own grief, but Gareth and his wife had to deal with the comments from other family members.

'We went to a wedding, our first event after her passing, and we were still in absolute shock – the grief was so real. We were standing talking, and Gareth ended up opening up and crying with a couple of friends. They were comforting him when his older brother walked over and said: "For fuck's sake – be a man! Pull yourself together and bloody get over it! Get on with your life!" In that moment his brother damaged Gareth's ability to feel, and Gareth shut down after that,' she said.

There is no shame in mourning, my Brothers, just as there is no shame in crying. Crying is as acceptable as laughing. Remember, it releases endorphins, which help us to feel better. Nobody has the right to ever tell you how to feel. Nobody.

Gareth threw himself into his work, and he wouldn't talk about his daughter at all. But by shutting down his emotions, he was also shutting out the one person who was experiencing the loss of her child, too – his wife.

'I would cry openly, and I would talk about her to anyone who wanted to hear. He became resentful that I could express my grief, that I was free to shed my tears, because he felt he couldn't do that. I longed for him to grieve with me, but he distanced himself in every way possible from my emotions.'

And, after 16 months, and the birth of another baby, their marriage was over.

'There was a gaping hole in our lives that my husband hadn't been able to adequately grieve the loss of. He had been shutting me out for over a year, coming home from work and going straight into the bedroom, where he would just go to bed, and shut the whole world out. I would try to encourage him to talk to me. I longed for him to open up, but he refused. He shut up and shut down. It was all too much. I wish another man in his life had given him the permission he needed to express his grief. The words of his brother were so harmful, even though I know he didn't intentionally mean to hurt him. They were brought up to never discuss their feelings or express themselves. I wish he had just put his arms around Gareth and told him then and there to cry as much as he needed.'

In our time of grief and sadness, the only thing that anyone ever wants is permission to feel how we feel, and be granted the space to share these emotions, however they look. Why should men keep their emotions in check? What is it about our society that we expect the strong, silent man to never express his feelings?

My Brothers, so many of you need to grieve the kinds of loss in your lives that you may never fully get over. There is no 'hardening up' to face your grief. That's not how this works. Grief is a process, and sometimes it is one with no immediate resolution.

This is okay.

The acceptance and the surrender of it being okay to feel the loss fully is really all I am able to do. I will always feel some sadness for my Mother, not just for my loss of her, but also because of how she lived her life.

It's not always death that causes our grief. Sometimes it's the abandonment of a parent. This can be just as hard in a different way - knowing that someone who should have loved you decided to leave you or withheld love from you. Sometimes it's even the loss of a relationship or a dream, or a physical ability.

My tall, strong, beautiful younger brother was diagnosed with heart failure in his early thirties. It was a huge adjustment for him to suddenly have none of the strength and physical stamina he was used to. He went from lifting weights at the gym and working at a job he loved to being bedridden or constantly exhausted, unable to do much at all. He completely lost the life he loved, and he's had to grieve the life he once knew and had, so that he can accept the life he has now.

I, too, have had to grieve the childhood I experienced, to be able to come to acceptance and live the life I have now. And when I say grieve, I mean cathartically release the pain of having a childhood that was filled with abuse.

I've met too many men whose grief has been unexpressed, and instead left to slowly rot away inside. However, it does eventually manifest itself - often in the form of rage, sickness, bitterness, anxiety or resentment. You can't let something rot inside you and not expect it to affect your life. It demands to be felt.

We must feel to heal.

Recently I was speaking with an 82-year-old retired psychotherapist named Graeme. Over the many years he had been practising as a therapist, he saw first-hand that there were three ways of expressing inner turmoil or pain, like grief. We either physically action it, through a form of addiction or violence; our body manifests it with sickness or a physical ailment; or we learn to action the distress or grief that we feel through our words.

So our options are: we harm ourselves or others, our body harms itself, *or* we learn to talk. Why is the talking bit so hard?

Graeme's Father taught him that feelings were dangerous, and because of this belief he didn't learn any 'feelings language' at all, so he could never express anything that went on inside of him. He hadn't been modelled this by his Father, and he hadn't been taught this anywhere else either. Because he, and many men like him, had no permission to feel anything, and no language to use, they understandably didn't know how to express what they were feeling.

How do you identify if you're feeling:

Fear	Not being heard	Humiliation
Frustration	Inadequacy	Grief
Disappointment	Rejection	Sadness
Abandonment	Shame	Trauma

What do they look and feel like to you?

Graeme said that this inability to express emotion was common among the majority of men in his generation, and that he ended up becoming a therapist himself, after a successful career as a scientist and a lecturer, so he could help men understand what was happening inside of them, and they could take the first step of getting in touch with their feelings, and be open with themselves.

Phil is another therapist I work alongside, hosting group therapy sessions from our barbershop. He told me that he has often found – in decades of working with men who struggle with violence and addiction – that grief has sat right under the anger. But for myriad reasons that grief wasn't allowed to be felt, so instead it manifested itself in adult years as violence. The grieving man has now become the angry man.

British author C. S. Lewis said: 'No one ever told me that grief felt so like fear.'

And this makes sense, too. Because it's hard to admit that we, as men, feel afraid. Society has told us for so long that we aren't allowed to feel afraid, because a 'real man' doesn't ever show fear or weakness, does he? Who decided that? Why do we allow that kind of unhealthy narrative of masculinity any kind of oxygen?

But first we need to distinguish destructive fear from constructive, useful fear. As we identified earlier, fear can perform a useful evolutionary function when it triggers a fight or flight response in us. It can energise us to identify danger and act in ways that will keep us safe and ready to fight another day. However, fear becomes problematic when it triggers an overreaction to an actual or perceived threat. And this often happens in situations where grief is involved. In these circumstances it can be hard for us to admit that there are things so far out of our control (for example in sickness and death) that we couldn't control them if we tried, with everything we have. It's hard to admit to not understanding loss and all it means. It's hard to surrender. It's hard to admit defeat as the tidal wave of grief washes over you.

But in these circumstances all I know about fear is that *it can lie*. Fear tells us we must be in control, so we scramble about in our need to make uncertain things certain. Fear keeps us bound. Fear tells us grief is weakness. Fear is tight fists clutching sand that manages to escape anyway.

Grief teaches us the power of love, and our resilience.

And love, my Brothers, is the exact opposite to fear.

Love is truth. Love is freedom. Love liberates.

Love can surrender and keep everything in an open palm, with arms wide open. Love tells us that nothing is ever really lost, so we don't have to be scared of saying 'Goodbye for now'. Love doesn't just say 'You can cry if you want' - it tells us loudly that **tears are welcome** and can be had wherever and whenever they're needed.

There is no fear where love resides.

Love accepts what is.

So grieve what you need to let go of for now, my Brothers. Sometimes it's okay if all you can do is breathe through the days, and find that those days turn into weeks and eventually years...

Cry your tears. Share your great and overwhelming sadness.

This grief just proves we have loved and that we are alive.

CONSIDER THE FOLLOWING tools from HelpGuide: Psychiatrist Elisabeth Kübler-Ross identified the five stages of grief you can find yourself going up and down or through at any stage. They are:

- Denial: 'This can't be happening to me.'

- Anger: 'Why is this happening to me? Who is to blame?'

- Bargaining: 'Make this not happen, and in return I will ...'

- Depression: 'I'm too sad to do anything.'

- Acceptance: 'I'm at peace with what happened.'

There is no one 'right' way to deal with grief, but you can try the following:

1. Acknowledge your pain.

2. Accept that grief can trigger many different and unexpected emotions.

3. Seek out face-to-face support from people who care about you.

4. Support yourself emotionally by taking care of yourself physically.

5. Recognise the difference between grief and depression.

Chapter twenty-one

She is not your excuse

ARE EXCUSES ONLY FABRICATED illusions we create to rationalise our behaviours when we're too afraid to go after what we really want?

The thirteenth-century Persian poet Rumi thought so, and I've sat with that idea for a while now. Me, a twenty-first-century barber, sitting with the concept that fear is beneath all my excuses. I asked myself what I'm afraid of, because the distance between any man and the life he says he wants tends to be excuses. And even between a man and the behaviour he says he *wants* to change, there tend to be excuses. The thing is, on the flip side of that fear is success – if only we can get out of our own way.

There are many reasons for the multiple circumstances and situations in our lives, but there should be no excuses from any adult in full ownership of their own life. We all know that person with every excuse under the sun. At any given moment they shift blame onto whoever is around. It is never their fault. It is never their responsibility. They take no ownership for any failing or setback. They can do no wrong because they cannot live with having to face the inevitable consequences of their decisions.

We could all justify or excuse our own poor behaviour and lack of action. I know how easy it is to play the victim card, and bleat 'poor me!' at any given moment, but this is only the child within us who hasn't yet matured, who would love to remove any sense of it being up to us to change something, or apologise for anything.

The child within us who refuses to grow up will always rather it was someone else's fault, because then they don't have to do any of the work required to change anything. We can sit there and repeat our sad story, with our starring role as the victim, and hope (at best) that someone feels sorry enough for us to rescue us, or pities us enough to collude with our excuses – which thousands of rescuers and enablers do around the world daily, in a variety of relationships.

But should anyone – even the significant woman in our life – have to rescue us from the inevitable consequences of the decisions we make? Can anyone else really be an Excuse?

AND IT WAS ALWAYS someone else's fault for a barber who once worked for me. He got caught stealing at the barbershop. Unfortunately, it wasn't the first time. I have had previous staff stealing from me, which is always a hard and awkward situation to face. But when I caught him red-handed stealing one day, I decided not to fire him on the spot, but to confront him face-to-face, and call him forward. When I did this, his immediate reaction was to blame his partner.

'I'm under too much pressure from the Missus with the bills!' he said.

I enquired what bills he was referring to, even though there was no justifiable excuse for him to take something that didn't belong to him.

'Just rent, and she's accounting for every dollar. I don't get any of my own money to myself with her budget.'

In that moment I'll admit that I honestly felt fucked off.

'Really?' I said. 'You really think that having to pay your

portion of the rent to your partner, who shares those expenses with you to cover your own living costs, justifies you to then steal off *me*? You realise we *all* have to pay to live, right? That's just reality for everyone, unless you are a child. If you want to make more money, then you'll need to consider working more, or cutting back in areas where you waste money, like the amount you smoke or drink.'

He said nothing. I think he realised his excuses didn't go down with me at all. I refused to be part of the drama he created, and regularly tried to drag other people into. I refused to excuse his bad behaviour, and I wondered if I was one of the few in his life who did this. We'll get back to him in a minute.

I wish I could tell you that he's the exception and not the rule, but, sadly, in my time as a barber I think I have heard probably every excuse for why someone is living a life they don't want – and most of the time the blame is shifted to either their partner, their parents, or even their children. There is no end to blame – it also goes on and on, to teachers, bosses, exes, colleagues and even neighbours. It even moves wider, to the government. Excuses and blame-shifting stop only when someone has the insight and the courage to take accountability.

In my 2019 TEDx talk *The Barbershop Where Men Go to Heal*, one of the key points I tried so hard to communicate was: **Your childhood trauma may not have been your fault, but your healing now is your responsibility.**

I make this particular point the heart of all my work, whether in my barbershops, or men's prison programmes, or in my advocacy against domestic violence – because, in all honesty, there are so many traumatised men among us. Men who did absolutely nothing to deserve the abuse or the pain inflicted on them when they were a vulnerable child.

So, Brothers, please hear me when I say that I do not minimise your suffering. I do not believe there are *ever* any acceptable excuses as to why people commit horrific acts against the children they should love, nurture and protect. I am so deeply sorry for your hurt. Please understand that when I invite you to take responsibility for your own healing and take accountability for your own life, I am *not* diminishing your story in the slightest, nor condoning whatever happened to you.

I am only asking you to consider how you really want the rest of your life to go. Do you want the same narrative of victimhood you have always had, or do you want to create a *new story*? One where you are not a victim, and where you need not shift blame to others. One where you have the courage to surrender the excuses, and start to live in a life that you are wholeheartedly part of, and accountable for.

How? I hear you ask me.

It actually comes down to our language, Brothers.

We start with how we think, and how we react to situations, and how we talk – to ourselves and to others.

Are our words bringing life to our situation? Do our excuses really take us further along in our own life, or do they continue to pull us down into the same spiral of self-destruction we've always known, and subconsciously believe is all we deserve? Do we unknowingly self-sabotage our own happiness with our excuses?

The barber who I caught stealing certainly did. Yes, he had a traumatic past. Yes, he had suffered sexual abuse as a child. Yes, he'd done extensive prison time for convictions stemming from a previous gang life. Life hadn't been easy at all, and hadn't dealt him the best cards, but the thing is – *now* he was in a good situation. He had a loving partner, and beautiful children who he had every opportunity to reconnect with. He also had a job with so much possibility, and a genuinely loving, supportive group of Brothers to live life with.

So how exactly did his past ruin his present? Honestly? With his excuses.

Excuses that, in his own mind, would explain and justify his poor behaviour. For me, the worst part of watching him on this path of self-destruction was seeing all the people who would collude with his bullshit excuses. They probably thought they were supporting and helping him. But, believe me, it never helped him once. It never gave him the life he said he wanted, or the life I believe he deserved.

When he got caught cheating on his partner with a client's

wife, he quickly brought it back to him being abused by a woman in his adolescent years. Therefore this was why he disrespected women now, he said. He just couldn't help it.

When he got hit up by his ex for child support - by the woman who had held it down alone with his child while he was incarcerated - he made an excuse of needing time to get his life sorted. Why couldn't she just understand, and give him the space he needed to sort things? This was more than a year after he had started working for me. In this year he'd turned down extra hours, and spent a good portion of his income every week on cigarettes and alcohol, but still didn't pay a cent of child support.

When he got caught repeatedly lying to his friends - people he called Brothers and considered family - he made the excuse of not knowing how to live truthfully because for too long he had been surrounded by dishonest people. 'It's just easier to lie and hide,' he said. 'I don't mean to - it just happens because it's now a habit I just can't break!'

When he came to work, down in the dumps one day following a heated argument he'd had with his partner, he blamed the entire situation on her: 'It started with her laziness. She didn't have my clothes clean for work. Then she was angry with me and went off because I asked her why she didn't do it. She has such a smart mouth, I'm not used to being spoken to like this, and now she's ruined my day and it's affecting how I talk to my clients!'

I had to eventually let him go when his stealing got so much out of control that he did it in front of other staff. He also blamed me for not paying him enough. According to him, it was my fault that I fired him for stealing from me, even though when I let him go it hurt me more than he could have imagined. I didn't want to let him go because I saw so much good in him. I saw the potential of the man he was born to be. Underneath the excuses and the lying and stealing was a great man who sold himself short in most moments of his life. His excuses stood between him and his own greatness.

So what do I say to a man whose whole life was not his responsibility, and who constantly relinquished all accountability?

I don't say much, but I do ask plenty:

If not now, when, Brother?

If you don't want to take responsibility now for the life you live, when do you plan to?

Do you realise that shifting blame from you to whoever becomes your newest scapegoat only ever renders you powerless in your own life?

Do you really want to be powerless and be this eternal victim?

Are you willing to forever make excuses for situations you could choose to take accountability for, and therefore grow and better yourself in?

Are you willing for your excuses to always outweigh your potential, and stop any future opportunities that could come your way?

Is this really the life you want?

AND AT THAT POINT, I will honour his sovereignty enough to respect whatever answers he gives me, because my deepest desire for him to live up to his potential is never, ever going to be bigger than any of his excuses. It just can't be.

Until *he* wants a life where he doesn't let his excuses rule his life, he will never have the life he could be living.

Please consider this in any relationship you have with someone who shifts blame or continually makes excuses. You cannot choose differently for them. You can't want more for them than they want for themselves.

No one else can help us more than we can help ourselves.

It really does start with us.

Our life truly begins when our desire for growth (which fundamentally comes from accountability and responsibility) outweighs all the excuses we carry.

To those of you who collude in the delusion of excuses, and make excuses for others' behaviour, can I gently ask you to consider why?

- Why do you believe that the natural course of action and consequence can be overruled in their case?

- Why do you believe that you have to eat up their excuses, and then make those same excuses for them to others?

- Why is it your job to protect anyone from consequences?

- If you would stop excusing/condoning/justifying their bad behaviour, what would happen – to you *and* to them? What would your relationship look like now?

There is nothing quite as empowering as fronting up to the right question. When something doesn't go the way I planned, or I feel I have failed in an area, I take time to reflect on what has happened. I no longer take the default response, using a victim mentality of blaming someone else, or making excuses.

Always pause to **reflect** instead of jumping to **react**.

Challenging myself internally with empowering questions automatically **moves me from a victim mentality to a growth mindset**. These days I'm able to do this in every area of my life, at any time. I can do this in my relationship with my wife in times of disagreement, in my role as a Father with my children when I feel the dynamics aren't as positive as I would like, in my friendships whenever there is conflict, and in my business when challenges inevitably arise.

I usually start with these questions:

HOW DID WE GET HERE?
This question gets me to really think about the overall situation, and how my beliefs have shaped my role in the situation. It allows me to consider the other person's beliefs, too. When we seek to genuinely understand something, with no hidden agenda or needing to be right, I find understanding usually comes. From understanding the situation, I can then move to the next question with greater clarity.

WHAT COULD I DO DIFFERENTLY, KNOWING WHAT I UNDERSTAND NOW?

Perspective is everything. This gives me the room to grow myself. If I made excuses, and refused to take this view, I would be robbing myself of growth. No amount of pride or ego is ever worth that, Brother.

Cancel excuses. Ask yourself questions instead, and when you have the honest answers within yourself, you will know what to do differently.

May you each have the courage to challenge yourself, and to grow. Your higher self and elevated consciousness depends on this.

Once the excuses stop, the life you say you want truly begins.

An invitation to heal

WHEN I SIT AND VISUALISE all the men who have ever graced my barbershop and sat in my chair, or worked alongside me, I know - without doubt - that my life is richer for each one of them. In our countless conversations, debates, tears, laughs and moments shared together, I am always so moved at **what genuine connection really does**.

True connection taught me.
True connection changed me.
True connection grew me.
True connection healed me.
True connection created Brotherhood.

THIS COMMUNITY OF BROTHERHOOD is my greatest career highlight as a barber. In my barbershop, with all kinds of men I call my Brothers, I have healed and have been privileged to witness the evolution of so many who society would easily discount and dismiss. I'm here to tell you that healing is possible because I've seen it be possible – numerous times, when the conditions were not really optimal.

I've watched men heal right before my eyes.

I've watched men rebuild from places of ruin.

I've watched men become the Fathers they have never, ever experienced themselves.

I've watched men leave metaphorical and physical prisons and step into freedom.

WHILE WE ARE MORE alike than we are different, and while I am no expert in anything beyond giving the dopest fade, I know from deep in my soul that the journey of healing is as unique as we are.

There is no one-size-fits-all approach, there are no magical bullet-point lists, nor is this book my invitation for you to cut and paste my story onto your own. I speak only from my own lived experience, with hope that it provides a window to another possibility of life – and I invite you, too, to own your story also, because in owning it there lies *our power* to transform our suffering, to redeem our pain, and to eradicate the great master of shame that I know once controlled every element of my life.

The invitation I share is available to my Usos (Brothers) who are incarcerated in institutions that do not prioritise genuine rehabilitation, the Usos who come from hoods like mine, with everything stacked up against them, and even to those Usos who live in material privilege, with access to everything – so much so that they can cover up their pain professionally.

The invitation of acknowledging the pain inside of you is for all, and the invitation of accepting responsibility for your healing is for all, too.

She is *not* your rehab – because our rehab is actually the space we create and gift ourselves with our willingness to own our story, heal our trauma and create a completely different way of living.

I wrote this book for every kid living, or having lived, in a home of violence and abuse.

I wrote it for the kids who have had all of their dreams kicked out of them.

I wrote our story to remind myself of what's possible, lest I ever forget – and to encourage each of you to believe that it's possible to re-write the narrative.

It's possible to eventually be everything we never got.

I'm living proof that a suicidal kid raised in a state house by immigrant parents, who lived in violence and abuse for the first 15 years of my life, can dream of being something else . . .

And then actually *be* something else.

We can break cycles.

We can heal.

And so we will.

And so we are.

Mauri ora whānau.

Fa'afetai tele lava.

Dear Mama, may your memory inspire a revolution.

Acknowledgements

Before anyone else, I want to acknowledge my siblings. George, Angus, Paulo, Faamanu, Vaosa, Tomai, Selafina and Katherine: those who know my story in ways no one else ever will. O uo mo aso uma, a o uso mo aso vale. No matter the distance, I love each of you.

To all our extended aiga and whānau: I can't list you all, but it goes without saying that blood knows blood and spirit knows spirit. I would, however, like to give my deepest thanks and honour to my dear Uncle: the beautiful Pastor Taimalelagi Sonny Papali'i Taimalelagi, who so graciously walked alongside our aiga in the passing of our Mum. Alofa atu nei. Alofa mai taeao Uncle.

To every single barber who has worked alongside me at My Fathers Barbers, from all the way back when we were just hanging in the barber shed in the hood till now: you have collectively gifted me lessons I carry into every space I walk in. I love and thank each of you.

To each of the barbers and stylists from around the world who have attended a hui, workshop or class of mine: thank you for doing this work daily in your own communities. You're changing the world, one head at a time!

To every 'client' who became a Brother: it's our conversations I hold close. Thank you for trusting me with your hair and your hearts.

To the men behind the wire and in our group therapy sessions: I see you all and remind you that while we are breathing, redemption is always possible. Ngā mihi Rachel Leota for the honour of being a patron at Corrections for Cohort 58. A special thank you to Anaru Paynes at Pathway for allowing me to hold space with our men at Christchurch Men's Prison, Auntie Lani Kouka and those who care for our rangatahi at the youth justice residence Te Puna Wai ō Tuhinapo with such compassion, and to Nicky Perkins and the whole whānau at Te Whare Manaakitanga at Rimutaka prison – this book's cover is dedicated to you.

To the many healers, teachers, mentors, spiritual leaders, kaumātua, advocates and therapists I have shared space and time with on my own healing/learning journey: I humbly thank you for all you've taught me with deep alofa to Kathi Harris, David Riddell, Phil Siataga, Nicky Sofai, Nu Telea, Patrick Te Wake, Ruru Harepeka Nako Hona, Sam Chapman, Thomas Wynne, Lino Hola, Luke Heka, Richie Steward, Conrad Fitz-Gerald, Ati Kurtulus Atligan, Ken Fale, Darrin Lyons, Josh Lamonaca, Gabrielle Bundy Cooke, Mary Ruston, Joanne Clark and a special thank you to Dr Elizabeth Mati from Le Va for making time for this book.

To the whole team at Penguin Random House New Zealand: thank you for believing in our story before it even was a story. Rachel Eadie: you helped birth our fourth baby - we love you! Thank you to Claire Murdoch for Mum's video, and to our beloved editor Sonia Yoshioka Braid - you walked this path with us with such care and kindness in such a hard time after Mum passed - fa'afetai, our Japanese sister! To Louisa Kasza, Katrina Duncan and Carla Sy: thank you for being part of this journey with us.

To Teresa Pomeroy and the whole It's Not OK team in Wellington: words fail me, fa'afetai tele lava. Special love for our kind, wise 'Auntie' Zaffa Christian, who has supported our mahi and journey with such genuine awhi, along with your sidekicks Joshua Peauafi, Brian Gardner, Scott Waring-Flood and Julie Anne Garnons-Williams. We love and appreciate you all so much.

To John Leonard and Catherine Savage at IHI Research, along with Hēmi Te Hēmi: we appreciate the way in which you took such care and understanding while researching and evaluating our mahi.

We are honoured to be ambassadors and to officially support the important work of the It's Not OK campaign (from the Ministry of Social Development), Aviva (in Christchurch), and MATE at Griffith University (as part of the Violence Prevention and Research team on the Gold Coast, Australia). We are always better together.

To friends who became Usos over the years: Josh Koia, John Cole, Sala Tiatia, Phil Borell, Albert Wilson, Sio Lealiifano, Jared Yeoward, Kenyon Clarke, Komene Kururangi, Dietrich Soakai, Maki Fonoti, Gareth Fraser, Garrick Cooper, Danny Yeoward, Peleti Oli, Lance Liufau, Luke Koia, Nasir Sobhani, Jayde Rangi Wilkinson, Brad Stent, Samuel Manu, Lio Fasi, Josh Waretini, Ash Vale, Anton Matthews and Joel Bell: I thank you for having my back and being in my corner. Each of you has in some way supported me, the mahi, my business, aiga and kaupapa. I value each of you and our kōrerō over the years immensely.

To my sisters by choice: Rochelle Cole, Negeen Sanaei, Trina Watkin, Tessa Apa, Charlotte Clarke, Lyren Fraser, Jade Moana, Fay Walker, Emma Fale, Danette Aperahama-Tiatia, Gina Eparaima, Sharon Malietoa, Sela Faletolu-Fasi, Theresa Taimalie-Pouvi, Ronda Shaskey, Hannah Chapman, Courtney Manu, Kaila Colbin, Eti Wilson, Jonique Oli and Tania Herbert. Your contribution to my life, and the life of my wife, and this work, will never be forgotten.

To Mark Tawha: you've impacted my life and work in ways no one else has. Thank you for gifting me with your vulnerability and story. I treasure this and you, my Uso. Forever your Brother.

To our biggest support and whānau – my toko Peni Likio and sissy Ngaroma Crown along with Nova and Tamāio: we couldn't and wouldn't ever want to do our life without you. Always got you. We love you, we like you, we life you.

To my Fathers: Paul Jamieson, thank you for first investing into my barbering career all those years ago. Armand Crown, thank you for choosing my wife how no one else ever had. Faamanu Brown, despite it all, I love and forgive you, Dad.

To my wife: there are no words in poetry or literature that'll ever express my gratitude for your love and friendship, but let me say this: the way you truly see me and walk alongside me is grace defined. Your gentle accompaniment in this healing song inspired lyrics of freedom I only visited in sleep. Till time engraves my final face, may your love forever engrave this heart where our children's children will echo your touch to the world as you touched mine.

To my three verses of this pese (song): Oceana, Angelou and Frida. Thank you for turning a sad song into a happy one. You were always my biggest invitation to do the work and heal. Always show up for each other and forever love the bridge to this song that brings us together, your beloved Mother.

I hope you'll always be proud to call me Dad.

Quotations

Page 33: adapted version of 'Transforming Pain' from *A Spring Within Us: A book of daily meditations* by Richard Rohr (CAC Publishing: 2016), pages 199, 120-121, © CAC, used by permission of CAC. All rights reserved worldwide.

Page 72: from *Dare to Lead: Brave work. Tough conversations. Whole hearts.* By Brené Brown (Ebury Publishing: 2018).

Page 94: from 'Dr Gabor Maté on Childhood Trauma, The Real Cause of Anxiety and Our "Insane" Culture', *Human Window* (humanwindow.com/dr-gabor-mate-interview-childhood-trauma-anxiety-culture/).

Page 94: from Dr Nicole LePera (the.holistic.psychologist) on Instagram.

Page 95: from *The Betrayal Bond: Breaking free of exploitive relationships* by Patrick Carnes (Health Communications Incorporated: 2019).

Page 116: from *The Dalai Lama Book of Quotes* by Travis Hellstrom (Hatherleigh Press: 2016).

Page 157: from *The Will to Change: Men, masculinity, and love* by bell hooks (Washington Square Press: 2004), page 120.

Page 157: from *All About Love: New visions* by bell hooks (HarperCollins: 2001), page 4.

Page 170: from *All About Love: New visions* by bell hooks (HarperCollins: 2001), page 9.

Page 186: from *Conversations with Maya Angelou* by Jeffrey M. Elliot (Virago: 1989).

Page 300: from *A Grief Observed* by C.S. Lewis (Faber & Faber: 2012).

Resources

She Is Not Your Rehab
For all official merchandise and enquires
Website sheisnotyourrehab.com
Instagram @sheisnotyourrehab
Facebook facebook.com/sheisnotyourrehab

It's Not OK
Family violence information line
Phone 0800 456 450
Website areyouok.org.nz

Need To Talk?
Counselling helpline
Phone 1737 (free to call or text any time)
Website 1737.org.nz

Safe To Talk
Sexual harm helpline
Phone 0800 044 334 or text 4334
Website safetotalk.nz

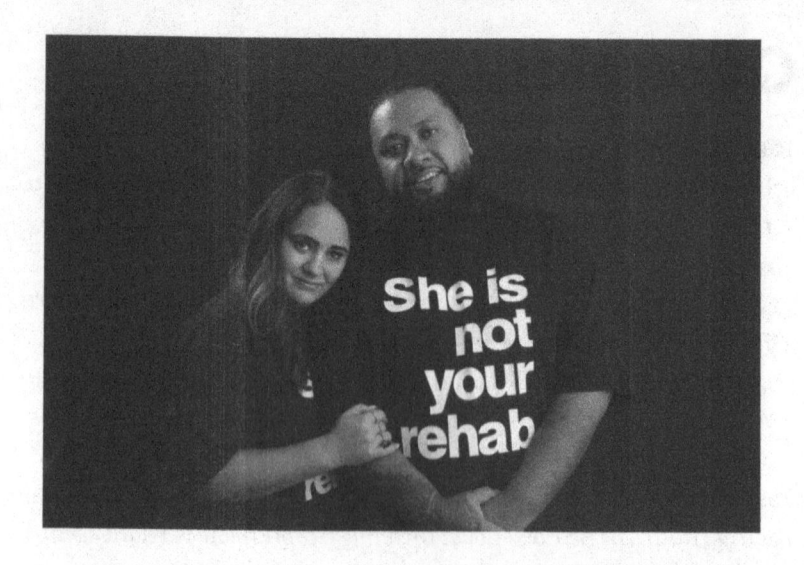

Mataio (Matt) Faafetai Malietoa Brown is an internationally acclaimed barber and hair artist and the founder of My Fathers Barbers, the barbershop where men go to heal.

His dedication to reviving the craft of barbering has seen him teach and demonstrate all over the world. While he's cut everyone from All Blacks to members of Wu-Tang Clan, Matt believes his true calling is his work to redefine society's view of masculinity – and to help end the cycle of domestic violence affecting families throughout the world.

Matt, a New Zealander of Sāmoan descent, together with his wife Sarah (Ngāpuhi/Te Rarawa), founded the anti-violence movement She Is Not Your Rehab (sheisnotyourrehab.com). In 2019, he outlined their kaupapa in a powerful TEDx Talk that continues to inspire today.

Matt collaborates with community and government organisations in New Zealand and abroad and hosts a men's group from his barbershop, enabling men to access free anti-violence therapy and support. He is the creator and facilitator of a barbering programme taught in men's prisons throughout New Zealand and a Corrections NZ patron. He is also an ambassador for the It's Not OK campaign with the Ministry of Social Development. He was a 2020 Westfield Riccarton Local Hero and a finalist for the Kiwibank New Zealand Local Hero of the Year award.

Matt and Sarah are proud parents to three and reside in Christchurch, New Zealand.